SURGICAL

Structured Answer and Essay Questions

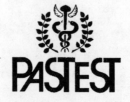

PASTEST

Dedication

In memory of our fathers

SURGICAL FINALS

Structured Answer and Essay Questions

Ramanathan Visvanathan BM FRCS
*Consultant Surgeon, Bronglais General Hospital, Aberystwyth,
Lately Honorary Senior Lecturer in Surgery
St Bartholomew's and the Royal London
School of Medicine and Dentistry
and Assistant Director, Professorial Surgical Unit,
St Bartholomew's Hospital, London*

John S P Lumley MS FRCS
*Professor of Surgery, St Bartholomew's and
the Royal London School of Medicine and Dentistry
and Honorary Consultant Surgeon
St Bartholomew's Hospital, London,
Member of Council, Royal College
of Surgeons of England,
Past World President
International College of Surgeons*

© 1997 PASTEST
Knutsford
Cheshire
Telephone: 01565 755226

First edition 1997

ISBN: 0 906896 69 X

A catalogue record for this book is available from the British Library.

Typeset by EDITEXT, Padfield, Nr Glossop, Derbyshire.
Printed by Hobbs the Printers Limited, Totton, Hampshire.

CONTENTS

PREFACE

With the current trend away from traditional essay questions for determining clinical knowledge, more and more examining bodies are introducing structured answer questions (SAQs) into undergraduate and postgraduate medical examinations. SAQs are designed to test problem-solving and decision-making in a structured and objective fashion, and are proving a reliable means of assessing knowledge and understanding in clinical practice.

In countries where medical education is in English, but one or more native languages are used for everyday communication, the introduction of SAQs is particularly welcome, since candidates are no longer penalised for an inability to write good English prose. Many busy examiners also appreciate the fact that SAQs can be marked more quickly, more easily and often more accurately than essays.

The aim of this book is to expose the reader to surgical SAQs but also to incorporate traditional essay questions.

Section I consists of SAQs based on the undergraduate clinical syllabus. The reader is encouraged to write his or her answers in the boxes provided so that marks can be accurately allocated.

Section II contains model answers and marking schedules for every question. The authors have also included short comments to expand on each topic and to highlight common pitfalls that should be avoided.

Section III offers advice on how to approach essay questions with a selection of structured outlines to teach good essay planning technique, and several complete genuine sample essays complete with illuminating examiners' comments.

Section IV contains a selection of typical questions to provide invaluable essay writing practice.

The three appendices to the book contain additional material likely to be helpful to the reader. Appendix A is an analysis of the final examination in surgery which explains the evolution of assessment techniques and may also be useful to senior doctors who are involved with setting examinations.

Appendix B provides the reader with the opportunity to sit mock SAQ examination papers. Each paper provides an authentic mixture of examination topics. Appendix C groups the essay questions in Section IV into mock exam papers.

This book is not intended as a comprehensive surgical text, but the range of questions provides a broad base for revision purposes. It may be used as a learning aid, together with surgical texts and other information sources, and it is also a valuable method of self-assessment enabling the reader to check his or her progress at each stage of the surgical course.

Acknowledgement

We wish to thank Yvonne Mallett for typing the drafts of the text, and Freydis Campbell and Jane Bowler, our publishers, for their support.

REVISION CHECKLIST

Use this checklist to record your revision progress. Tick the subjects when you feel confident that you have covered them adequately. This will ensure that you do not forget to revise any key topics.

Chapter 1: Surgical Physiology
☐ Fluid and electrolyte therapy
☐ Acid-base balance
☐ Enteral and parenteral feeding
☐ Transfusion reactions

Chapter 2: Trauma and Burns
☐ Head injury assessment
☐ Cervical spine injury
☐ Thoracic injury
☐ Blunt abdominal trauma
☐ Fracture of pelvis and long bones
☐ Assessment of burns
☐ Colloid and crystalloid therapy in burns

Chapter 3: Orthopaedics
☐ Osteoarthritis of the hip
☐ Rheumatoid arthritis
☐ Osteomyelitis
☐ Bone tumours
☐ Kyphoscoliosis

Chapter 4: Neurosurgery
☐ Head injury
☐ Meningomyelocoele
☐ Hydrocephalus
☐ Hypothalamic/pituitary lesions
☐ Peripheral nerve injuries

Chapter 5: Eyes, ENT and Skin
☐ The painful red eye
☐ Retinoblastoma
☐ Glaucoma
☐ Uveitis
☐ Nose bleed
☐ Chronic sinusitis
☐ Otitis media

- ☐ Tonsillitis
- ☐ Melanoma
- ☐ Squamous carcinoma
- ☐ Basal cell carcinoma

Chapter 6: Endocrinology, Breast and Chest Diseases
- ☐ Toxic goitre
- ☐ Thyroid malignancy
- ☐ Parathyroid hyperplasia
- ☐ Cervical adenopathy
- ☐ Adrenal tumours
- ☐ Benign breast disease
- ☐ Nipple discharge
- ☐ Breast cancer
- ☐ Lung cancer
- ☐ Lung abscess
- ☐ Coronary bypass surgery

Chapter 7: Upper Alimentary Tract
- ☐ Tongue lesions
- ☐ Salivary gland lesions
- ☐ Oesophageal stricture
- ☐ Peptic ulcer disease
- ☐ Gastric cancer
- ☐ Splenomegaly

Chapter 8: Liver, Gall Bladder and Pancreas
- ☐ Cirrhosis and portal hypertension
- ☐ Gall bladder: inflammation and stones
- ☐ Obstructive jaundice
- ☐ Pancreatitis

Chapter 9: Small and Large Bowel
- ☐ Bowel obstruction including hernia
- ☐ Appendicitis
- ☐ Ischaemic bowel
- ☐ Peritonitis
- ☐ Colonic polyps and cancer
- ☐ Inflammatory bowel disease
- ☐ Perianal lesions

Chapter 10: Urology
- [ ] Renal tumours and stones
- [ ] Bladder tumours and stones
- [ ] Urinary retention and incontinence
- [ ] Prostatic enlargement
- [ ] Testicular tumours
- [ ] Urethral stricture

Chapter 11: Vascular Surgery
- [ ] Carotid artery disease
- [ ] Cervical rib syndrome
- [ ] Aortic aneurysms
- [ ] Acute and chronic lower limb ischaemia
- [ ] Lower limb amputation
- [ ] Varicose veins
- [ ] Deep venous thrombosis

ABBREVIATIONS

ABG	Arterial blood gases estimation
AXR	Abdominal X-ray (antero-posterior)
BP	Blood pressure
Ca^{++}	Calcium ions
CL^-	Chloride ions
CO_2	Carbon dioxide
CT	Computerised tomogram
CVP	Central venous pressure
CXR	Chest X-ray
ERCP	Endoscopic retrograde cholangio pancreatogram
ESR	Erythrocyte sedimentation rate
FBC	Full blood count
FNAB	Fine needle aspiration biopsy
H^+	Protons or hydrogen ions
H_2O	Water
Hb	Haemoglobin
HCO_3^-	Bicarbonate ions
hr	Hour
ICP	Intra-cranial pressure
INR	International coagulation ratio
IV	Intravenous
IVU	Intravenous urography
K^+	Potassium ions
kcal	Kilocalorie
KCl	Potassium chloride
kg	Kilogram
l	Litre
LFT	Liver function test
ml	Millilitre
Mg^{++}	Magnesium ions
MRI	Magnetic resonance imaging
Na^+	Sodium ions
NaCl	Sodium chloride
O_2	Oxygen
OGD	Oesophago–gastro–duodenoscopy
PCV	Packed cell volume
PO_4^{---}	Phosphate ions
PTA	Percutaneous transluminal angioplasty
U&E	Urea and electrolytes
U/S	Ultrasound scan
WBC	White blood count

RECOMMENDED READING LIST

General surgical texts
Clinical Examination of the Patient
Lumley JSP and Bouloux PMG, Butterworth Heinemann, 1994.
This book, with 486 colour photographs, serves as a useful guide for formulating and perfecting examination techniques.

An Introduction to the Symptoms and Signs of Surgical Disease
Browse N, 2nd edition, Edward Arnold, 1991.
This is a very good guide to surgical examination technique and differential diagnosis of common signs and is also very useful for reference.

Lecture Notes in General Surgery
Ellis H and Calne R, 8th edition, Blackwell Scientific, 1992.
In this text, each surgical disease is classified with useful sections on pathology and management. This is especially helpful for learning how to write structured essay plans.

Surgical Diagnosis and Management: A Guide to General Surgical Care
Dunn DC and Rawlinson JN, 2nd edition, Blackwell Scientific, 1991.
This well-structured text strikes a balance between explaining general principles and giving practical details for the day-to-day management of surgical patients (e.g. when drains and sutures come out). It is particularly useful on the wards in the final year and during the house job.

Spot Diagnosis in General Surgery
Ellis H, 2nd edition, Blackwell Scientific, 1993.
A collection of colour photographs of patients, pathology specimens and X-rays. Each picture is accompanied by background information and relevant questions. A useful revision aid for the clinicals and orals.

Oxford Handbook of Clinical Surgery
McLatchie GR, Oxford University Press, 1990.
This pocket handbook is useful for carrying on the wards. It is full of management plans and practical procedures. However, there is not much explanation of basic principles and, although structured, the format is not consistent. It should not be mistaken for a basic surgical text.

Pocket Examiner in Surgery
Northover J and Treasure T, 2nd edition, Churchill Livingstone, 1996.
This pocket book is full of questions and answers and is very useful for carrying on the wards and clinics and quizzing each other.

Essential Surgery: Problems, Diagnosis and Management
Burkitt HG, 2nd edition, Churchill Livingstone, 1995.
A popular textbook of general surgery aimed at clinical students. Its main advantages are its very readable style, clear explanations of the pathophysiological basis of surgical problems and illustrated synopses of the main stages of common surgical operations.

Bailey and Love's New Short Practice of Surgery
Mann CV, Russell RCG and Williams NS, 22nd edition, Chapman & Hall, 1995.
A complete reference textbook that forms the basis of surgery after the Finals.

Orthopaedic texts
Essentials of Orthopaedic Examination
Hammer A, 3rd edition, Edward Arnold, 1994.
A small, clearly illustrated book which adopts a systematic approach to its examination schemes.

Physical Signs in Orthopaedics
Klenerman L and Walsh HJ, BMJ Publishing Group, 1994.
Over 200 black and white photographs with questions and answers. A useful revision aid for the clinicals.

Clinical Orthopaedic Examination
McRae R, 3rd edition, Churchill Livingstone, 1990.
A good guide to examining orthopaedic patients. Each step in the examination schemes is clearly illustrated with line drawings.

Concise System of Orthopaedics and Fractures
Apley AG and Solomon L, 2nd edition, Butterworth Heinemann, 1991.
A standard orthopaedics book, full of useful sketches, photographs and X-rays which bring the text to life. It contains examination schemes for different joints.

HOW TO USE THIS BOOK

This book consists of four sections. Sections I and II contain structured answer questions (SAQs) and answers. Sections III and IV contain essay questions and model answers.

Write your answers to the SAQs in the boxes provided. When you have finished, turn to Section II to mark your answers. Allow half marks for incomplete answers, and full marks for sensible and accurate alternatives that the authors have not considered. We hope that the examiners are equally understanding.

Every answer includes a short section of comments which provide concise teaching notes on each topic. Where necessary, refer to the list of recommended textbooks for further information.

At the back of the book, appendices B and C contain typical examination papers enabling you to gain experience of working under timed conditions. Twelve SAQs or four essay questions constitute a two-hour written paper.

Use the Revision Checklist provided to monitor your progress by ticking off subjects with which you feel confident.

SECTION I:
STRUCTURED ANSWER QUESTIONS

CHAPTER 1: SURGICAL PHYSIOLOGY

Question 1

A 78-year-old man weighing 53 kg was admitted from a nursing home with a 14-day history of persistent vomiting. He was very dehydrated and malnourished.

(a) (i) How would you estimate his fluid and electrolyte deficit? (1 mark)
 (ii) List the fluid and electrolyte preparations you would use, with their approximate compositions, to correct his deficit. (2 marks)
 (iii) How would you monitor his fluid replacement therapy? (2 marks)

(b) (i) How would you assess his state of nutrition? (2 marks)
 (ii) Discuss briefly how you would work out his protein and calorie requirements. (3 marks)

Question 2

A 65-year-old man was admitted with a three-day history of vomiting. A diagnosis of gastric outlet obstruction was made. He was placed on nasogastric aspiration and an IV infusion of 5% dextrose, alternating with Hartmann's (Ringer lactate) solution over the next 48 hours. His serum biochemistry on admission was Na^+ 120 mmol/L; K^+ 3.7 mmol/L, HCO_3^- 40 mmol/L. His urinary pH at the end of this period was 7.2.

(a) (i) State the biochemical diagnosis on admission. (1 mark)
    (ii) Comment on the fluid and electrolyte replacement that followed. (3 marks)

(b) Write a note on the metabolic factors responsible for the production of acidic urine. (6 marks)

Question 3

A 60-year-old man underwent elective abdominal surgery for repair of an aortic aneurysm.

(a) (i) What is the metabolic response in respect to fluid and electrolyte balance in the first 24 hours of surgery? (2 marks)
   (ii) How would you adjust the fluid and electrolyte requirements during this period? (2 marks)

(b) His urine output fell to below 30 ml/hr following surgery.
   (i) How would you determine the cause of his oliguria? (4 marks)
   (ii) What remedial measures would you take? (2 marks)

Question 4

An adult male undergoing abdominal surgery became pyrexial and developed an erythematous skin rash during a postoperative blood transfusion.

(a) (i)   What factors are involved in these reactions? (2 marks)

      (ii) What measures would you take to counteract these complications? (2 marks)

(b) In the post-operative period the patient required a 10-unit blood transfusion.

      (i)   What is the effect of this transfusion on liver function and clotting factors? (2 marks)

      (ii) What is the effect on plasma potassium and calcium levels and how would you achieve homeostasis of these ions in the plasma? (4 marks)

Question 5

A 34-year-old man with advanced infection with the human immunodeficiency virus (HIV) developed bowel obstruction which required emergency surgery.

(a) (i) State the measures taken to protect theatre personnel from accidental inoculation with the patient's body fluids with regard to wearing of protective garb. (2 marks)

    (ii) What important measures should be taken with regard to safety in surgical instrument usage? (3 marks)

(b) (i) List the changes in the haematological or biochemical parameters that would, in the perioperative period make him susceptible to haemorrhage. (2 marks)

    (ii) List the haematological or biochemical changes in the perioperative period that would make him susceptible to infection. (3 marks)

Question 6

A 43-year-old woman suffering from diabetes mellitus was admitted as an emergency with gangrene of the toes of her left foot. ABG estimation revealed a pH of 7.1 and a partial pressure of CO_2 of 6.8.

(a) (i) State the acid-base disorder present. (1 mark)
     (ii) Give two causes for this. (2 marks)

(b) (i)   State the further investigations you would request. (3 marks)
     (ii) How would you manage the metabolic disorder? (4 marks)

Question 7

A 49-year-old man with a malignant stricture of the oesophagus had lost 20% of his normal body weight over a three-month period.

(a) (i) State the cause of his weight loss. (1 mark)
    (ii) How would you categorise his nutritional state? (1 mark)
    (iii) List two clinical findings that would reflect the nutritional state. (2 marks)

(b) (i) How would you improve his nutritional state? (3 marks)
    (ii) How would you monitor your nutrition therapy? (3 marks)

Question 1

A 30-year-old man was brought to the Accident and Emergency department having sustained a closed head injury from a blow to the back of the head.

(a) How would you assess the level of consciousness? (2 marks)

(b) List the physical signs you would elicit to establish the extent of the intracranial injury. (3 marks)

(c) (i) List the types of intracranial bleeding that may be present and state one investigation that would demonstrate the lesion. (2 marks)
     (ii) Write a short note on your management. (3 marks)

Question 2

A 23-year-old motorcyclist sustained chest injuries in a road accident and was airlifted to the Accident and Emergency department.

(a) State your immediate measures to assess and maintain respiratory and circulatory function. (3 marks)

(b) Identify two immediately life-threatening intra-thoracic emergencies during your primary clinical survey. (2 marks)

(c) (i) Write a note on the management of an open chest wound. (2 marks)
    (ii) Write a note on the management of an haemo-pneumothorax. (3 marks)

Question 3

A driver of a motor vehicle involved in a head-on collision with another vehicle was air-lifted to the Accident and Emergency department fully conscious and communicative but becoming increasingly breathless, with central cyanosis and bruising over his right upper chest.

(a) (i) State the two probable causes for his progressive respiratory failure. (2 marks)

    (ii) List the clinical signs you would elicit to confirm your diagnoses. (2 marks)

(b) (i) State one blood investigation you would urgently request. (1 mark)

    (ii) State the radiological investigations that would confirm the diagnosis. (1 mark)

(c) State four potentially lethal thoracic injuries he may have sustained which may not be apparent during the initial clinical survey. (4 marks)

Question 4

A 43-year-old woman fell off her horse in a riding accident. She complained of severe and persistent upper abdominal pain radiating to her back.

(a) (i)   List the possible intra-abdominal visceral injuries sustained. (2 marks)
    (ii)   State one non-invasive investigation you would perform to assess the presence and extent of an intra-abdominal injury. (1 mark)

(b) (i)   How would you monitor this patient in the Accident and Emergency department? (2 marks)
    (ii)   What are the immediate resuscitatory measures you may be called upon to perform? (2 marks)

(c) Discuss the clinical and other findings that would require an emergency surgical exploration of the abdomen. (3 marks)

Question 5

You are a member of an air ambulance team attending to a 28-year-old man with multiple injuries at the site of a road traffic accident.

(a) State in order of priority your measures to ensure patient survival until transfer to a trauma centre. (5 marks)

(b) The patient is trapped in the wreckage of his vehicle and his transfer is delayed by three hours. Discuss your supportive measures. (3 marks)

(c) List the ideal composition of an air ambulance team. (2 marks)

Question 6

An 18-year-old motor cyclist involved in a road traffic accident was admitted to the Accident and Emergency department. He was fully conscious but complained of severe neck pain.

(a) List the possible injuries to the cervical spine and cervical cord he may have sustained. (3 marks)

(b) When gently examining the neck:
  (i)   What findings would suggest a spinal injury? (1 mark)
  (ii) What manoeuvre should you not perform? (1 mark)

(c) If he were found to have a spinal fracture and cord lesion at C5–T1 level:
  (i)   Discuss your treatment of the injury. (2 marks)
  (ii) How would you prevent complications as a sequelae to the injury? (3 marks)

Question 7

An 8-year-old girl suffered hot water scalds to the whole of her chest and abdomen. She was admitted to the Accident and Emergency department conscious and very distressed.

(a) (i)   How would you estimate the surface area affected? (1 mark)
     (ii) State the immediate medical measures you would take. (4 marks)

(b) (i)   How would you distinguish between a partial and a full thickness skin burn? (2 marks)
     (ii) How would you calculate the fluid replacement for the first 24 hours? (3 marks)

Question 8

A 30-year-old secretary was rescued from an office fire. She was breathless and coughing, with traces of soot around her nose and mouth. She had suffered no external burns.

(a) (i)   State the injury sustained. (1 mark)
     (ii) Give your immediate resuscitation measures. (2 marks)

(b) She develops stridor and respiratory distress.
     (i)   State the pathological process involved. (2 marks)
     (ii) How would you manage her airway? (2 marks)
     (iii) How would you treat the injury sustained? (3 marks)

Question 9

A 20-year-old man injured his neck when the scrum collapsed on him while playing rugby.

(a) (i) How would you avoid compounding a suspected spinal injury? (2 marks)
   (ii) How would you investigate for the integrity of the cervical spine? (2 marks)

(b) If the patient is unconscious list the clinical findings that suggest a cervical cord injury. (3 marks)

(c) Write a note on neurogenic shock following cervical cord injury. (3 marks)

Question 10

A 15-year-old boy was admitted to the Accident and Emergency department following a traffic accident. He was conscious but very pale, with bruising over the right lower chest and abdomen, and a swelling of the right thigh and knee.

(a) How would you assess for the following:
  (i) Lung injury. (2 marks)
  (ii) Intra-abdominal injury. (2 marks)
  (iii) Lower limb injury. (2 marks)

(b) He was developing hypovolaemic shock. List your immediate measures to resuscitate him. (4 marks)

Question 11

A 5-year-old boy was seen in the Accident and Emergency department, having sustained hot water scalds to his arms, chest and abdomen at home.

(a) How would you determine on examination the extent and depth of his wounds? (3 marks)

(b) State your criteria for admission. (3 marks)

(c) Write a note on the methods of dressing his wounds. (4 marks)

Question 12

A 38-year-old railway worker was admitted to the Accident and Emergency department with electrical burns to his back and arm, from contact with high tension overhead conductors.

(a) State three urgent priorities in his clinical assessment. (3 marks)

(b) Write a note on the type of burn injury sustained. (3 marks)

(c) Discuss the effect of the injury on the heart, kidneys, skeletal muscle and nervous system. (4 marks)

Question 13

A 49-year-old motorist sustained burns to 35% of his body surface from burning fuel in a traffic accident.

(a) How would you estimate his fluid requirements for the first 24 hours? (3 marks)

(b) What measures would you take to prevent wound infection? (4 marks)

(c) How would you manage a non-survivable burn injury? (3 marks)

CHAPTER 3: ORTHOPAEDICS

Question 1

A 9-year old schoolgirl was seen at the orthopaedic clinic with a 4-month history of pain in her left groin and hip, and a progressive limp. She had no history of trauma or other symptoms.

(a) List the positive findings you would expect on examining her hip.
(3 marks)

(b) (i) State two diseases that may present thus at this age. (2 marks)
    (ii) List the radiological features you would expect to see in each. (2 marks)

(c) What are their complications if left untreated? (3 marks)

Question 2

A 17-year-old schoolboy sustained an external rotational injury to his right ankle during a rugby tackle. There was considerable pain, bruising and swelling.

(a) List the possible injuries to the ankle. (4 marks)

(b) Radiology of the ankle and distal tibia and fibula showed no fracture. What related bony and/or ligamentous injuries would you wish to exclude? (2 marks)

(c) Write a note on the treatment of an unstable ankle injury. (4 marks)

Question 3

A 40-year-old woman suffered with pain, swelling and loss of mobility in her fingers, which over a period of time affected her wrists and feet.

(a) (i) State the likely diagnosis. (1 mark)
     (ii) Write a note on the pathological changes in the joints. (3 marks)

(b) List the positive blood investigations in this disease. (3 marks)

(c) State the principles of management. (3 marks)

Question 4

A 64-year-old woman with pain, stiffness and limitation of movement in her left hip was diagnosed as having osteoarthritis.

(a) List the radiological features in the hip joint. (3 marks)

(b) State non-surgical measures to alleviate symptoms and preserve function. (3 marks)

(c) (i) List the indications for operative treatment. (3 marks)
     (ii) State the operation of choice for this patient. (1 mark)

Question 5

A 6-year-old boy sustained a supracondylar fracture to his right arm during a fall in the school playground.

(a) Write a note on your management. (4 marks)

(b) Eight hours after the fracture was reduced the child was crying with severe pain and was unable to grasp objects with the right hand. The forearm was swollen and the radial pulse absent. Write a note on your diagnosis and treatment. (3 marks)

(c) List the complications of this fracture. (3 marks)

Question 6

(a) Write a note on how you would diagnose and treat congenital dislocation of the hip in the neonatal period. (5 marks)

(b) List the factors which give rise to this condition. (2 marks)

(c) If the diagnosis is delayed until the child starts walking, discuss the treatment options and prognosis. (3 marks)

Question 7

A child of 5 years presented to her family practitioner with a 3-day history of severe pain in her left forearm, with fever and malaise. The forearm was inflamed and swollen.

(a) (i) State the probable diagnosis. (1 mark)
     (ii) Write a note on the investigations that would aid the diagnosis.
          (3 marks)

(b) Give three differential diagnoses of the forearm swelling. (3 marks)

(c) Outline your treatment. (3 marks)

Question 8

A boy of 8 years was referred from a child welfare clinic with a growth curve well below the normal range. Clinically there was thickening of his wrists and ankles, and bowing of his legs.

(a) (i) State the likely clinical diagnosis. (1 mark)
   (ii) List the radiological features which would confirm your diagnosis. (2 marks)
   (iii) List the biochemical features which would confirm your diagnosis. (2 marks)

(b) (i) State the causative factors. (3 marks)
   (ii) Outline the treatment. (2 marks)

Question 9

A 60-year-old man presented with long-standing dull pain in his back and hips, and was found to be of short stature, with kyphosis of the spine and slight forward bowing of his legs.

(a) (i) State the probable clinical diagnosis. (1 mark)

   (ii) Discuss the bony changes that characterise this disease. (4 marks)

(b) List four complications of this disease. (2 marks)

(c) Write a note on the principles of treatment. (3 marks)

Question 10

A 47-year-old factory worker presented with a painless, fluctuant swelling in his right groin. A kyphotic angulation of the dorsal spine was observed on examination.

(a) (i) State the probable diagnosis. (1 mark)
    (ii) Discuss the pathological basis of the clinical findings. (2 marks)

(b) List the investigations to confirm your diagnosis. (3 marks)

(c) (i) Discuss your objectives in treatment. (3 marks)
    (ii) State a serious complication that may be precipitated in this patient. (1 mark)

Question 11

A 5-year-old child suffering from protein-calorie malnutrition presented with an inflamed, swollen and painful forearm of four days' duration.

(a) (i)   State two lesions that may present thus. (2 marks)

    (ii) How would movements in that limb be affected? (2 marks)

(b) (i)   List the common organisms that are implicated. (2 marks)

    (ii) Discuss the treatment of these two lesions. (4 marks)

Question 1

An 11-month-old male infant was referred to the Neurosurgical Clinic with a history of failure to thrive and achieve milestones. A progressive increase in skull circumference had been noted since birth.

(a) (i) State the likely diagnosis. (1 mark)
    (ii) What are the positive clinical findings? (2 marks)
    (iii) State one important investigation to confirm your diagnosis. (1 mark)

(b) (i) State a common cause for this condition. (1 mark)
    (ii) Give two associated malformations of the central nervous system. (2 marks)

(c) Write a note on the definitive treatment for this condition. (3 marks)

Question 2

A woman with a nine-month history of epileptic fits and headaches was found to have focal neurological signs and papilloedema.

(a) (i)   State your working diagnosis. (1 mark)

     (ii) Discuss briefly the pathophysiology of the abnormal findings. (3 marks)

(b) (i)   State two investigations that would reveal the lesion. (2 marks)

     (ii) Why would a lumbar puncture be contraindicated? (1 mark)

(c) List three benign and three malignant lesions that would present thus. (3 marks)

Question 3

A previously healthy 32-year-old woman was admitted complaining of sudden onset of severe headache, with nausea and vomiting. She was found to be drowsy with neck stiffness.

(a) (i) State the likely diagnosis and the underlying lesion. (2 marks)
     (ii) If her condition deteriorates, state the progressive changes in the clinical findings. (3 marks)

(b) (i) State one non-invasive investigation to confirm your diagnosis. (1 mark)
     (ii) State your findings on lumbar puncture. (1 mark)

(c) Write a note on the medical and surgical principles of her management.
(3 marks)

Question 4

A conscious 75-year-old woman was admitted with a left hemisphere stroke.

(a) (i)   List three prime neurological findings. (2 marks)

      (ii) List four risk factors of stroke. (2 marks)

(b) The patient's condition deteriorates; outline your immediate management. (6 marks)

Question 5

A 6-year-old child presented with fever and fits. A cranial CT scan revealed a brain abscess.

(a) How would you arrive at this diagnosis clinically? (3 marks)

(b) (i)   List four causative organisms. (2 marks)
     (ii) List two underlying sources of infection that predispose to brain abscess in this child. (2 marks)

(c) Write a note on specific treatment. (3 marks)

Question 6

A 56-year-old woman complained of gradual onset of pain in her neck, radiating down her left arm. She also experienced tingling down the limb during neck extension.

(a) List three lesions of the spinal cord and three lesions of the cervical spine that may give rise to her symptoms. (3 marks)

(b) Write a note on the likely neurological findings. (3 marks)

(c) (i) List the radiological investigations to confirm your diagnosis. (2 marks)
    (ii) State the principles of treatment. (2 marks)

Question 1

A 70-year-old woman suffered a sudden painless loss of vision in one eye.

(a) Give four possible causes. (4 marks)

(b) State three associated systemic diseases. (3 marks)

(c) If she had suffered loss of vision in both eyes, state two probable causes. (3 marks)

Question 2

A 3-year-old toddler was seen in the Accident and Emergency department with a 5-day history of a painful red eye.

(a)   List four possible causes. (2 marks)

(b)   Write a note on your examination of the eye. (4 marks)

(c)   If a white pupillary reflex was seen on fundoscopy, state your probable diagnosis and management. (4 marks)

Question 3

An 11-year-old boy was admitted with right-sided proptosis, oedematous conjunctivitis (chemosis) and reduced visual acuity. He was found to be pyrexial, dehydrated and lethargic. There was a recent history of recurrent acute sinus infection.

(a) (i) State your clinical diagnosis. (1 mark)
    (ii) What microbiological and radiological investigations would you request? (2 marks)

(b) (i) State your medical management of this condition. (2 marks)
    (ii) How would you monitor the response to your medical measures? (2 marks)

(c) The child failed to improve, with deterioration in his eye signs. A CT scan showed right purulent pansinusitis and an abscess under the orbital plate of the ethmoid bone.

(i) State the surgical measures required. (2 marks)

(ii) State a potentially lethal complication of this condition. (1 mark)

Question 4

A cricketer fielding close to the wicket was struck in the orbit by a firmly hit cricket ball. He presented to the Accident and Emergency department with periocular ecchymosis and periorbital swelling.

(a) (i) State the probably orbital injury sustained. (1 mark)
    (ii) State the mechanism of the injury to the orbit. (2 marks)

(b) (i) Discuss the positive findings when examining for orbital damage. (3 marks)
    (ii) List the investigations you would require to exclude bony injury. (1 mark)

(c) Discuss the principles of managing this injury. (3 marks)

Question 5

A 48-year-old man presented to the ENT clinic with a six-week history of progressive hoarseness not responding to antibiotics.

(a) List four non-malignant lesions of the vocal cords that may present thus. (2 marks)

(b) Write a note on two methods of clinically examining the larynx. (4 marks)

(c) A biopsy of a small lesion on the vocal cord revealed a squamous cell carcinoma (glottic carcinoma). Discuss the treatment options available. (4 marks)

Question 6

A 5-year-old boy was referred from the pre-school clinic with a persistent hearing loss in one ear. A diagnosis of 'glue ear' was made.

(a) (i) Discuss the nature of the hearing loss. (2 marks)
    (ii) List three predisposing factors. (2 marks)

(b) Describe the appearance of the ear drum in this condition. (2 marks)

(c) Discuss two methods of surgically treating this condition. (4 marks)

Question 7

A 54-year old woman presented with a 12-week history of a circumscribed 2.5cm diameter itchy, ulcerating pigmented skin lesion on her upper back; it had recently bled.

(a) (i)   What are the other clinical features of the lesion you would look for on examination? (1 mark)

      (ii) State a malignant lesion that may present thus. (1 mark)

      (iii) How is it staged histologically? (2 marks)

(b) How would you treat this lesion? (3 marks)

(c) Write a short note on the public health measures you would adopt to reduce the incidence of this form of skin cancer in the community. (3 marks)

Question 8

A small, circumscribed raised lesion on the cheek of an 87-year-old woman bled following minor trauma.

(a) State three malignant lesions that may present thus. (3 marks)

(b) If your clinical diagnosis is a form of skin cancer, what are the treatment options available? (4 marks)

(c) (i) Discuss the association of solar radiation with the development of skin lesions. (2 marks)
    (ii) What protective measures would you advise? (1 mark)

CHAPTER 6: ENDOCRINOLOGY, BREAST AND CHEST

Question 1

A 35-year-old woman presented to the surgical clinic with a gradually enlarging asymptomatic swelling in the front of her neck.

(a) (i) State the structures likely to be involved. (2 marks)
    (ii) How would you clinically distinguish one from the other? (2 marks)

(b) Discuss the investigations you would perform to confirm your clinical impression. (2 marks)

(c) If you had diagnosed a goitre, state the clinical findings that would require surgical intervention. (4 marks)

Question 2

A 30-year-old woman presents to the surgical clinic with symptoms of restlessness, insomnia and a preference to cooler weather. She has a pulse rate of 110 per minute and a painless swelling of her thyroid gland.

(a)   (i)   State your probable diagnosis. (1 mark)

      (ii)   List other clinical features that would support this diagnosis. (3 marks)

(b)   State the investigations you would perform to assess her thyroid function. (3 marks)

(c)   Discuss the management of this condition. (3 marks)

Question 3

A 64-year-old woman presented to the surgical clinic with a long-standing thyroid swelling, complaining of recent onset of pain in the neck and hoarseness.

(a) Write a short note on the clinical findings that would assist you in reaching a diagnosis. (3 marks)

(b) State the probable cause of the hoarseness and the examination you would carry out to confirm this. (2 marks)

(c) (i) State the investigations you would request to confirm your clinical diagnosis. (3 marks)
    (ii) What is referred to as a 'cold nodule' on thyroid imaging? (2 marks)

Question 4

A 46-year-old woman in chronic renal failure sustained a pathological fracture of her hip.

(a) Discuss briefly the metabolic basis for the fracture. (3 marks)

(b) Her serum parathyroid hormone (PTH) titres were raised. Explain the parathyroid hyperfunction in relation to renal failure. (3 marks)

(c) State how you would counteract the elevated PTH titres. (4 marks)

Question 5

A 25-year-old, otherwise healthy woman gave a 12-month history of headaches of increasing frequency, accompanied by flushes and sweats. Her BP was 180/120 on presentation. A CT scan of her abdomen revealed a right-sided adrenal tumour measuring 5.5 cm in size. Her 24-hour urinary metanephrines and vanillyl mandelic acid levels were significantly raised.

(a) (i) State the likely diagnosis. (1 mark)
    (ii) What other biochemical test(s) would confirm your diagnosis? (2 marks)

(b) (i) Discuss the functional disorders caused by this lesion (2 marks)
    (ii) Give the medical management of these. (3 marks)
    (iii) State the definitive treatment for this disease. (2 marks)

Question 6

A 58-year-old woman presented with a nine-month history of progressive fatigue, weight gain and spontaneous skin bruising. She was found to be hypertensive, with impaired glucose tolerance.

(a) (i) State the endocrine disorder. (1 mark)
    (ii) Name one laboratory investigation that would confirm your diagnosis. (1 mark)

(b) (i) State the source of this disease. (1 mark)
    (ii) Give one investigation to define the anatomical site of the lesion. (1 mark)
    (iii) List three other endocrine disorders that may arise from the same gland. (3 marks)

(c) Discuss the principles of treating this patient. (3 marks)

Question 7

A worried 46-year-old woman, attending the Breast Clinic as an urgent referral, gave a three-week history of a blood-stained discharge from her right nipple.

(a) (i) List three possible abnormal findings during your examination of her breast. (2 marks)

   (ii) List other anatomical regions you would include in your examination. (2 marks)

   (iii) List three clinical diagnoses you would consider. (3 marks)

(b) List three specific investigations that would assist you in arriving at a diagnosis. (3 marks)

Question 8

An anxious 36-year-old woman, attending the Breast Clinic as an urgent referral, gave a three-week history of an asymptomatic lump in her left breast.

(a) (i) List the clinical characteristics of the lesion you would assess. (2 marks)

(ii) State the sites of lymphatic drainage of the breast. (2 marks)

(b) List the investigations that would assist in confirming your clinical diagnosis. (2 marks)

(c) List the treatment modalities available for breast malignancy. (4 marks)

Question 9

A 78-year-old woman presented with an asymptomatic, hard and irregular mobile lump in her right breast.

(a) (i) State the most likely histological diagnosis. (1 mark)
   (ii) How would you assess distant spread? (3 marks)

(b) The lump has been present for over six years with little alteration in size
   (i) Is the diagnosis of malignancy still likely? (1 mark)
   (ii) How would you treat her if malignancy is confirmed? (2 marks)
   (iii) If she declines your offer of treatment, what would be the likely outcome? (3 marks)

Question 10

A 35-year-old woman was referred to the Breast Assessment Clinic following a community breast screening programme.

(a) State three investigations performed on a small, barely palpable breast lump. (3 marks)

(b) The lump was removed under stereotactic guidance and was found to be a lobular carcinoma with vascular invasion. List your investigations for the presence of distant metastases. (3 marks)

(c) State the principles of treatment. (4 marks)

Question 11

An 18-month-old boy presented with episodes of breathlessness and cyanosis, usually following feeds. On examination bowel sounds were heard over his left chest wall.

(a) (i)   State your working diagnosis. (1 mark)
    (ii) List the radiological findings on chest X-ray. (3 marks)

(b) List the complications of delayed diagnosis. (3 marks)

(c) State the principles of surgical treatment. (3 marks)

Question 12

A 46-year-old man gave a four-month history of cough and breathlessness, with right-sided chest pain. A thoracoscopy was arranged.

(a) Write a short note on this procedure. (3 marks)

(b) An empyema thoracis was diagnosed; state how you would manage this condition. (4 marks)

(c) List the aetiological factors associated with this diagnosis. (3 marks)

Question 13

A 71-year-old woman presented with an enlarged asymptomatic lymph node at the root of her neck.

(a) List four malignant diseases that may present thus. (2 marks)

(b) Biopsy of the node revealed a deposit of small cell carcinoma. State your clinical diagnosis and the investigations to confirm this. (4 marks)

(c) State the principles of surgical treatment of this lesion. (4 marks)

Question 14

A 69-year old pensioner suffered from angina of effort which had progressively worsened over a 20-month period despite medical measures to control his symptoms.

(a) (i)   State your probable diagnosis. (1 mark)

      (ii) State two non-invasive investigations to confirm your diagnosis. (1 mark)

      (iii) What information would be obtained therefrom? (2 marks)

(b) (i)   Write a note on the radiological method used to investigate and treat this disease. (3 marks)

(c) Write a note on the principles of surgical treatment of this disease.
(3 marks)

Question 1

A 40-year-old man presented to the surgical clinic with a two-year history of an asymptomatic, slow-growing firm lump on the side of his face just below the lobe of his ear.

(a) (i) State the likely diagnosis. (1 mark)

     (ii) List the characteristics of the lesion you would ascertain on examination. (3 marks)

(b) A request was made for cytological confirmation by percutaneous needle biopsy of the lesion. Give your comments. (2 marks)

(c) (i) Write a note on the principles of surgical treatment. (3 marks)

     (ii) What structures must be preserved from injury? (1 mark)

Question 2

A 29-year-old man was referred to the Accident and Emergency department with a 10-day history of progressive pain and swelling of his mouth and upper part of his neck. He was pyrexial, with inflamed palpable nodes in his neck.

(a) (i) State the likely diagnosis and the anatomic planes involved in the inflammatory process. (2 marks)
   (ii) List the pathogenic organisms that are associated with this lesion. (2 marks)

(b) (i) What are the consequences of progression if left untreated? (2 marks)
   (ii) How would you treat this lesion? (4 marks)

Question 3

A 71-year old man was referred to the surgical clinic with increasing difficulty in swallowing and significant weight loss over a period of six months.

(a) What other aspects of the history would assist you in arriving at a clinical diagnosis? (2 marks)

(b) (i) List the possible causes of dysphagia in this patient. (3 marks)
    (ii) Name two investigations which would confirm your clinical diagnosis; what information would you obtain from each? (2 marks)

(c) Write a note on the aetiological factors associated with any two diagnoses. (3 marks)

Question 4

A 40-year-old male business executive presents with a six-month history of upper abdominal pain that comes on in the evenings and wakes him up in the early hours of the morning. Symptoms are relieved by food, milk and antacids.

(a) (i) State your clinical diagnosis. (1 mark)
    (ii) Discuss briefly the aetiological factors that are associated with this disease. (2 marks)

(b) State one investigation that would demonstrate both the site and appearance of the lesion, and write a note on how this investigation is performed. (2 marks)

(c) (i) Discuss briefly the principles of treating this disease. (3 marks)

    (ii) List the complications of this disease. (2 marks)

Question 5

A 4-month-old infant was referred with a history of projectile vomiting and poor weight gain since birth. His mother had felt a lump in his abdomen following feeds.

(a) (i)   State your working diagnosis. (2 marks)

      (ii) List two differential diagnoses. (2 marks)

      (iii) What is the nature of the lump that the mother felt? (1 mark)

(b) Write a short note on the pathophysiology of this lesion. (2 marks)

(c) Discuss the principles of treatment. (3 marks)

Question 6

A newborn baby was found to regurgitate his feeds and developed a post-aspiration respiratory infection.

(a) (i) State your working diagnosis. (1 mark)
    (ii) State the radiological investigation required to confirm your diagnosis. (1 mark)

(b) (i) Write a note or illustrate the congenital malformations that may present thus. (4 marks)
    (ii) State a simple procedure that could be performed at birth to exclude this abnormality. (2 marks)

(c) What are the principles of treatment? (2 marks)

Question 7

A 34-year-old otherwise healthy woman gave a history of heartburn and belching with waterbrash.

(a) (i)   State your probable diagnosis. (1 mark)
      (ii) Write a short note on the underlying lesion. (3 marks)
      (iii) State one investigation you would perform to confirm your diagnosis.
         (1 mark)

(b) (i)   Discuss briefly the measures you would advise to alleviate her symptoms. (2 marks)
      (ii) State the surgical procedures that would effect a cure. (3 marks)

Question 8

A 39-year-old man with a six-month history of dyspepsia unresponsive to antacids was found to have an apparently normal gastric mucosa on endoscopy.

(a) List the tests you would perform on antral mucosal biopsies obtained in order to reach a diagnosis. (3 marks)

(b) (i) If a bacterial presence was detected, state the probable diagnosis. (1 mark)
    (ii) How would you treat this infection? (3 marks)

(c) Write a note on the association of this pathogen with lesions of the stomach and duodenum. (3 marks)

Question 9

A 38-year-old man was seen in the Accident and Emergency department vomiting blood. An emergency upper GI endoscopy revealed bleeding from oesophageal varices.

(a) How would you control the bleeding? (4 marks)

(b) State the pathophysiology of this condition. (3 marks)

(c) What would be your follow-up protocol on this patient? (3 marks)

Question 10

A 36-year-old woman on anti-inflammatory medication for symptoms of rheumatoid arthritis developed severe upper abdominal pain of sudden onset. She was found to be pyrexial with a rigid abdomen.

(a) (i) State the probable diagnosis. (2 marks)
(ii) List the radiological features to confirm your diagnosis. (2 marks)

(b) Write a note on your treatment measures, including surgical measures if appropriate. (4 marks)

(c) State your measures to prevent recurrence of this disease. (2 marks)

Question 11

A 32-year-old man underwent an elective splenectomy for hypersplenism.

(a) List the three main types of postoperative bleeding in this patient. (3 marks)

(b) How would you manage such a haemorrhage in the immediate post-operative period? (4 marks)

(c) State the factors that may increase his susceptibility to infections, and your preventive measures. (3 marks)

Question 12

A 76-year-old man complained of a sore tongue. On examination a 1 cm ulcer was present on the postero-lateral aspect on the tongue with a patchy, white hyperkeratotic discoloration of the surrounding mucosa.

(a) List the clinical findings that would suggest a malignant ulcer. (3 marks)

(b) What is the surrounding mucosal lesion called? List the aetiological factors associated with this lesion. (3 marks)

(c) The ulcer on the tongue was found to be a squamous carcinoma. Discuss the principles of treatment. (4 marks)

CHAPTER 8: LIVER, GALL BLADDER AND PANCREAS

Question 1

A 40-year-old housewife complains of severe right upper abdominal pain radiating to the back, two hours after eating fried food.

(a) (i)   Give your working diagnosis. (1 mark)

     (ii) Give three physical signs you would expect to support this diagnosis. (2 marks)

     (iii) Give one non-invasive investigation to support your diagnosis. (1 mark)

(b) Write a note on the pathogenesis of the disease. (3 marks)

(c) Discuss briefly the principles of surgical treatment. (3 marks)

Question 2

A 66-year-old woman with a history of calculus cholecystitis was admitted as an emergency feeling acutely ill, with progressive jaundice, right upper quadrant pain and rigors over the previous 3 days.

(a) (i)   State your probable diagnosis. (1 mark)
    (ii) Outline the causation and pathogenesis of this condition. (2 marks)
    (iii) State the immediate blood investigations you would request, giving the reason for each. (3 marks)

(b) State two non-invasive methods of visualising the biliary tree in order to confirm your diagnosis. (1 mark)

(c) Discuss the principles of treatment. (3 marks)

Question 3

A 34-year-old woman became progressively jaundiced immediately follow-ing an elective cholecystectomy.

(a) (i)   State the most likely cause of her jaundice. (1 mark)
     (ii) State an invasive investigation that would confirm your diagnosis.
           (1 mark).
     (iii) How would you prepare the patient for this procedure? (2 marks)

(b) She developed a tender abdomen with rebound, rigors and raised white
     blood. State your diagnosis. (2 marks)

(c) Write a note on the measures the surgeon should adopt to avoid these
     complications. (4 marks)

Question 4

A 38-year-old woman presented acutely with symptoms of small bowel obstruction. She gave a six-month history of fatty food intolerance and upper right-sided abdominal pain with mild episodes of jaundice.

(a) (i)   State the likely diagnosis. (1 mark)
    (ii) What is the pathogenesis of the disease? (1 mark)
    (iii) List the salient features on the plain abdominal X-ray. (2 marks)

(b) How would you treat her bowel obstruction? (3 marks)

(c) Write a short note on your management of the underlying pathology. (3 marks)

Question 5

A 48-year-old woman presented with severe upper abdominal pain and vomiting. On examination, her abdomen was rigid and tender. A plain erect abdominal X-ray was normal. Both serum amylase titres and white cell count were raised.

(a) (i) State the probable diagnosis. (1 mark)
    (ii) Give two main causes for this condition. (2 marks)

(b) Outline your management. (4 marks)

(c) List the complications of this disease. (3 marks)

Question 6

A 78-year-old man gave a six-week history of progressive jaundice, anorexia and weight loss. Clinically he was malnourished and pale, and abdominal examination revealed a palpable gall bladder and a liver edge.

(a)   State the probable diagnosis and list the investigations you would require to confirm it. (3 marks)

(b)   (i)   List your treatment options for this patient. (3 marks)
      (ii)   What factors would decide against major curative surgery? (2 marks)

(c)   If the patient underwent an abdominal operation, list the postoperative complications that are associated with jaundice. (2 marks)

Question 7

A 15-year-old boy was injured in a traffic accident and underwent surgical repair of a laceration to the right lobe of the liver.

(a) Postoperatively he vomited fresh blood.
    (i) State two possible causative factors. (1 mark)
    (ii) How would you treat these complications? (4 marks)

(b) The abdominal drain drained a clear fluid with a high amylase content.
    (i) State the significance of this finding. (1 mark)
    (ii) How would you identify the lesion? (2 marks)

(c) If the abdominal drain had drained bile instead.
    (i)   State the probable lesion. (1 mark)
    (ii) How would you define the lesion? (1 mark)

Question 8

A 30-year-old man presented to the Accident and Emergency department complaining of severe central abdominal pain and nausea of seven days' duration.

(a) In the absence of positive significant clinical findings a working diagnosis of acute non-specific abdominal pain was made.
   (i)   What do you understand by this statement? (1 mark)
   (ii) Give examples of psychosomatic states that may be associated with this presentation. (2 marks)

(b) Further enquiries revealed a history of alcoholism, with previous similar presentations to hospitals.
   (i)   State the probable diagnosis and the investigations required to confirm this. (3 marks)
   (ii) Write a note on the principles of treatment. (4 marks)

Question 1

A 3-month-old baby boy was referred to the Accident and Emergency department with a three-day history of fretfulness and colic. He had vomited bile-stained fluid the previous day and passed blood-stained mucus per rectum.

(a) (i) State the likely diagnosis. (1 mark)

(ii) Write a note on the factors that may be associated with this condition. (2 marks)

(b) What would be the findings on abdominal examination? (3 marks)

(c) (i) State one investigation that is used both to confirm the diagnosis and to treat the condition. (1 mark)

(ii) How is this procedure performed? (3 marks)

Question 2

A 69-year-old woman was referred to the surgical clinic with a three-month history of alteration in bowel habit, with intermittent passage of loose motions containing mucus and blood.

(a)   List the possible causes of her symptoms. (3 marks)

(b)   If dietary and infective causes are excluded, outline the specific measures you would adopt to arrive at a diagnosis. (4 marks)

(c)   If abdominal examination revealed hepatomegaly and ascites, state the further investigations you would request and the information obtained therefrom. (3 marks)

Question 3

A 59-year-old woman was admitted with a three-week history of progressively severe crampy lower abdominal pain and distension. She had not opened her bowels for the past 10 days, felt nauseated and had vomited twice over the previous two days.

(a) (i) State your expected clinical findings. (2 marks)
    (ii) What is your working diagnosis? (1 mark)

(b) (i) State one radiological investigation that would confirm your diagnosis. (1 mark)
    (ii) List the findings. (2 marks)

(c) State your initial management of this patient. (4 marks)

Question 4

A 45-year-old, 70 kg man was admitted with symptoms of acute small bowel obstruction.

(a) List the findings on abdominal X-ray which would confirm the diagnosis. (2 marks)

(b) (i)   How would you assess the accompanying fluid and electrolyte derangement? (3 marks)
     (ii) How would you treat it? (3 marks)

(c) If the obstruction is due to adhesions as a consequence of previous abdominal surgery, state your management. (2 marks)

Question 5

A 4-day-old neonate was seen in the Accident and Emergency department with progressive abdominal distension and not passing meconium since birth.

(a) List the causes of large bowel obstruction in the newborn. (2 marks)

(b) Rectal examination on this patient was followed by a spontaneous passage of a large quantity of meconium.
   (i)   State the probable diagnosis. (1 mark)
   (ii) Write a note on its pathogenesis. (3 marks)

(c) (i)   State two investigations to confirm your diagnosis. (2 marks)
   (ii) State the principles of surgical treatment. (2 marks)

Question 6

A neonate presented at birth with a defect in the abdominal wall, covered by a transparent sac containing loops of intestine. The umbilical cord was attached at its apex.

(a) (i) What is this condition called? (1 mark)
(ii) Write a note on the development of this anomaly. (3 marks)

(b) Write a note on the principles of treatment for this condition. (3 marks)

(c) List three malformations of the alimentary tract resulting in failure of canalisation of the lumen. (3 marks)

Question 7

A 43-year-old manual worker presented to the Accident and Emergency department with a four-day history of fever and a painful, tender, fluctuant swelling immediately lateral to the anus.

(a) (i)   State the probable diagnosis. (1 mark)
     (ii) Write a note on the evolution of this lesion. (3 marks)

(b) He was sent home on a course of antibiotics. Soon afterwards the swelling ruptured draining pus, and the pain and temperature settled. However, the wound continued to discharge intermittently over the next 3 months.
     (i)   State the complication that had ensued. (1 mark)
     (ii) How should his original lesion have been treated? (2 marks)
     (iii) Write a note on the principles of treating the current complication. (3 marks)

Question 8

A 35-year-old man was referred to the surgical clinic with a four-month history of painless rectal bleeding following defaecation.

(a) (i) How would you examine the ano-rectum to arrive at a diagnosis? (3 marks)
     (ii) List three diseases of the colon that may present thus. (3 marks)

(b) The patient also complained of an intermittent fleshy protrusion at the anus.
     (i) State the most likely cause. (1 mark)
     (ii) List three procedures used in treating this condition. (3 marks)

Question 9

A 68-year-old woman presented with a six-week history of tenesmus and the passage of blood-stained mucus in her motions. Examination revealed an ulcerating lesion in the rectum.

(a) (i) How would you characterise the clinical features of this lesion? (3 marks)

    (ii) State one investigation that is required to make a definitive diagnosis. (2 marks)

(b) A diagnosis of a rectal adenocarcinoma was made.

    (i) State the most frequent site of blood-borne metastases. (1 mark)

    (ii) What is your method of its detection? (1 mark)

    (iii) Write a note on the surgical treatment of this lesion. (3 marks)

CHAPTER 10: UROLOGY

Question 1

A 29-year-old man was referred to the Surgical Clinic with a six-week history of an asymptomatic swelling in the right side of his scrotum.

(a) (i)   State the structures that may be involved. (3 marks)
     (ii) Describe how you would, by examination, localise the lesion.
           (2 marks)

(b) (i) State three testicular tumours found in young adults. (3 marks)
     (ii) List the principles of treating testicular tumours. (2 marks)

Question 2

A middle-aged man was seen in the Surgical Clinic with an asymptomatic intermittent swelling in his right groin. He gave a 12-month history of nocturnal frequency and dribbling.

(a) State the nature of his groin swelling and examination findings that would support your diagnosis. (3 marks)

(b) State the probable cause of his urinary symptoms and discuss the relevant findings on examination. (3 marks)

(c) Discuss briefly the management of this patient. (4 marks)

Question 3

A 15-year-old boy presented to the Accident and Emergency department with sudden onset of severe pain in his left testicle two hours previously.

(a) (i)   State the likely diagnosis. (1 mark)
     (ii) State your findings in support of the diagnosis. (3 marks)

(b) Write a short note on your treatment. (3 marks)

(c) If the child presented 48 hours after the onset of symptoms, how would this alter your management? (3 marks)

Question 4

A 70-year-old man complained of passing bubbles of gas in his urine. Six months previously he had undergone surgical removal of a colonic tumour, followed by radiotherapy to the region.

(a) (i)   What is this symptom called? (1 mark)
     (ii) State two probable causes for this symptom. (2 marks)

(b) List the investigations that would confirm your diagnosis. (3 marks)

(c) List four other diseases that may produce this complication. (4 marks)

Question 5

A 75-year-old man is returned to the ward following transurethral prostatectomy.

(a) List the early and late complications of this operation. (4 marks)

(b) State two causes of prostatic enlargement that require prostatectomy. (2 marks)

(c) List the complications that may arise if symptoms of prostatism are left untreated. (4 marks)

Question 6

A 28-year-old man was referred to the urology clinic complaining of impotence.

(a) State three causes for this. (3 marks)

(b) Seminal fluid analysis suggested sterility. What criteria would this report be based on? (3 marks)

(c) (i) State a chronic infection that may produce sterility in this patient. (1 mark)
  (ii) How would you confirm your diagnosis? (3 marks)

Question 7

A 35-year-old man in end-stage renal failure underwent cadaveric renal transplantation. Post-operatively he remained oliguric.

(a) List four possible causes for the oliguria. (2 marks)

(b) Write a note on the investigations you would perform to arrive at a diagnosis. (3 marks)

(c) (i) State the drugs used for immunosuppression following transplantation. (2 marks)
     (ii) Write a note on the complications associated with their use. (3 marks)

Question 8

A 28-year-old woman was referred to the urology clinic with a three-month history of severe intermittent unilateral loin pain radiating to the groin, accompanied by nausea and vomiting.

(a) (i) State your clinical diagnosis. (1 mark)
     (ii) What immediate investigation would confirm your diagnosis at the bed side? (2 marks)

(b) Outline your management. (5 marks)

(c) List four predisposing causes. (2 marks)

Question 9

A 5-year-old boy presented to the paediatric surgical clinic with an incidental discovery of a left flank mass by his mother.

(a) (i) List four lesions of the kidney that may present thus. (2 marks)
     (ii) State three imaging procedures used to arrive at a diagnosis.
          (3 marks)

(b) If these investigations reveal a malignant tumour of the left kidney.
     (i) State three investigations required to determine the presence of
          distant metastases. (2 marks)
     (ii) Outline the three modalities of treatment. (3 marks)

Question 10

A 34-year-old otherwise healthy male presented with progressive symptoms of straining to void, with poor urinary stream and dribbling. An indurated area was palpable in the line of the penile urethra.

(a) State the probable diagnosis and list the probable causes of this condition. (3 marks)

(b) State the complications of this lesion. (3 marks)

(c) Write a note on the principles of treatment. (4 marks)

Question 11

(a) Define stress incontinence of urine and discuss its causes in a 35-year-old woman. (3 marks)

(b) How would you investigate her symptoms? (3 marks)

(c) State the principles of treatment. (4 marks)

Question 1

A 79-year-old man was admitted to the Accident and Emergency department with a four-hour history of sudden onset of severe pain and numbness in his left leg extending up to his mid-thigh.

(a) State your working diagnosis and the aetiological factors with which it may be associated. (3 marks)

(b) List the clinical findings in the limb supporting your diagnosis. (3 marks)

(c) Write a note on the treatment. (4 marks)

Question 2

A 68-year-old man complains of gradual onset of right calf claudication radiating up to his thigh on walking distances exceeding 75 yards.

(a) (i) State your likely diagnosis and the anatomic site(s) of his lesion. (2 marks)
     (ii) Write a short note on the disease process causing his symptoms. (3 marks)

(b) Give four common risk factors in this disease. (2 marks)

(c) What measures would you advise him to adopt to alleviate his symptoms, to stop progression of the disease and improve his walking distance? (3 marks)

113

Question 3

A 59-year-old woman complained of rest pain in her left foot keeping her awake at night. She also had difficulty in walking.

(a) List the clinical findings that would lead to a working diagnosis. (4 marks)

(b) (i) Name one radiological investigation you would request to demonstrate the lesion. (1 mark)
(ii) Write a short note on how radiological procedures may be used to treat her symptoms. (2 marks)

(c) Discuss briefly the surgical options available to relieve her symptoms. (3 marks)

Question 4

A 68-year-old man underwent a femoral arteriogram and balloon angioplasty for an external iliac arterial stenosis.

(a) List the symptoms and clinical findings that would have led to this procedure. (3 marks)

(b) Soon afterwards he complained of severe pain in the limb, which had become blanched and pulseless.
   (i) State two likely causes for this complication. (2 marks)
   (ii) State your management. (3 marks)

(c) List the risk factors in the development of peripheral vascular disease. (2 marks)

Question 5

A 76-year-old man presented with a pulsatile swelling in his right groin three days after a coronary angioplasty, where access was gained via the right femoral artery.

(a) (i) State the most likely diagnosis. (1 mark)
     (ii) State one non-invasive investigation for confirmation. (1 mark)
     (iii) How would you treat this? (2 marks)

(b) The patient developed a cold, painful and pulseless lower limb immediately after the coronary angioplasty.
     (i) State two probable causes. (2 marks)
     (ii) How would you treat each of these complications? (4 marks)

Question 6

A 75-year-old man was referred to the surgical clinic with an incidental finding of a palpable, pulsatile and expansile upper abdominal mass of approximately 10 cm in diameter.

(a) (i) State the likely diagnosis. (1 mark)
    (ii) Discuss the pathological changes that produced this lesion. (2 marks)

(b) State one non-invasive investigation you would request to identify the anatomical limits of the lesion. (1 mark)

(c) (i) Write short notes on the principles of surgical treatment of this patient. (3 marks)
    (ii) Write short notes on the pre-operative preparation of the patient. (3 marks)

Question 7

A 64-year-old man was admitted to the Accident and Emergency department complaining of severe back pain, radiating to the left loin accompanied by nausea and feeling faint. He was found to be hypotensive, with a rapid pulse.

(a) (i) State your clinical diagnosis. (1 mark)
    (ii) Outline your resuscitatory measures. (3 marks)

(b) State the surgical treatment for this condition. (1 mark)

(c) (i) If he were on long-term warfarin therapy for atrial fibrillation and his INR was found to be over 4.0, what would be your diagnosis? (2 marks)
    (ii) State your specific treatment measures. (3 marks)

Question 8

A 70-year-old pensioner gave a history of dizzy spells over an eight-month period. More recently he experienced occasional blurring of vision, with transient loss of vision in his right eye.

(a) (i)   Give the probable cause of his symptoms. (1 mark)
     (ii) State the underlying factors that may be causative or associated with his disease. (2 marks)

(b) (i)   Name one invasive investigation to confirm your diagnosis. (1 mark)
     (ii) What information would you obtain therefrom? (2 marks)

(c) Write a note on your proposed treatment. (4 marks)

Question 9

A 50-year-old woman with a long history of progressively symptomatic lower limb varicosities bled profusely from a chronic leg ulcer. She presented to the Accident and Emergency department with a tourniquet applied to control the haemorrhage.

(a) Write a note on the pathogenesis of the ulcer and the bleeding therefrom. (3 marks)

(b) Comment on the method used for haemostasis and state how you would control the bleeding. (3 marks)

(c) Discuss her management once haemostasis has been achieved. (4 marks)

Question 10

A middle-aged woman was seen in the surgical clinic with a long history of a painful ulcer over the medial aspect of her left ankle, with swelling of the foot. She also complained of long-standing varicose veins in that limb.

(a) (i) State the type of ulcer and its cause. (1 mark)
     (ii) Comment on the characteristics of the lesion and the state of the surrounding skin. (2 marks)

(b) (i) Write a short note on the measures you would adopt to bring about the healing of the ulcer. (2 marks)
     (ii) How would you prevent its recurrence? (1 mark)

(c) State two other types of chronic leg ulcers and discuss their pathophysiology. (4 marks)

Question 11

A 46-year-old woman who had undergone abdominal surgery five days previously developed pain and cramps in her left calf and lower thigh.

(a) Discuss the clinical findings you would elicit in order to arrive at a diagnosis. (3 marks)

(b) (i) State a diagnosis which carries potentially lethal complications. (1 mark)
    (ii) Write a short note on the pathophysiology of this condition and its complications. (3 marks)

(c) Write a short note on the management of this patient. (3 marks)

Question 12

A 35-year-old woman who had been discharged from hospital two days previously, following abdominal surgery, developed sudden chest pain, with shortness of breath.

(a) (i) What is the most likely diagnosis? (1 mark)
     (ii) State the two most important investigations to confirm your diagnosis. (2 marks)

(b) Discuss the treatment for this condition. (5 marks)

(c) List the preventive measures to avoid this complication. (2 marks)

SECTION II:
SAQ MODEL ANSWERS

CHAPTER 1: SURGICAL PHYSIOLOGY

Answer 1

(a) (i) Thirst; skin turgor; BP (postural drop); serum urea and electrolyte measurement; urine output

1

(ii) N/saline, 5% & 10%; dextrose 1.8% or 3.0% dextrose in normal saline; Hartmann's solution; KCl solution (amount in mmols to be carefully titrated against daily or twice daily serum levels)

2

(iii) CVP monitoring; 3-hourly urea and electrolyte estimation; hourly urine output; daily Hb and PCV estimation; daily weighing of patient

2

(b) (i) Hb, PCV, serum albumin, folate, B12, Fe; skinfold thickness by use of callipers

2

(ii) Daily calorie and nitrogen requirements are calculated on the ideal weight for the patient's height and body build. Energy requirements vary from 1500 to 3000 kcal per day and are provided by administered carbohydrate 40% and lipid 60%. Daily nitrogen requirement is based on replacing existing protein depletion and on-going breakdown in wear and tear. In hypercatabolic states this amounts to 0.25 to 0.39 kg of nitrogen

3

Comment

Calories are provided by carbohydrate and fat. They should be in proportion to the nitrogen intake in the ratio of 150 kcal to 1 g of nitrogen. Administered nitrogen should not be used as an energy source, as it would perpetuate the state of negative nitrogen balance. The patient receiving 2000 kcal would require 13 g of nitrogen daily. Vitamins and trace elements are essential as dietary supplements for normal metabolic function and must be included in feeding regimes.

Answer 2

(a) (i) Metabolic (hypokalaemic, hyponatraemic, hypochloraemic) alkalosis

1

(ii) The fluid regime did little to correct the Na^+ and K^+ ion
     loss in vomit and gastric aspirate

(b) Gastric outlet obstruction leads to loss of water, Na^+, K^+ and
    H^+ ions. Anti-diuretic hormone production is stimulated, and
    aldosterone production is suppressed by the hypothalamus.
    This results in renal tubular resorption of Na^+ and K^+ ions at
    the expense of H^+ ions, which produces an acid urine, thereby
    exacerbating the metabolic alkalosis

6

Comment
The inappropriate production of acid urine in metabolic alkalosis
is due to renal tubular response to dehydration and low serum $[Na^+]$
by resorption of Na^+ and excretion of H^+ and K^+ in order to maintain
trans-cellular ionic equilibrium. Counteractive measures should
replace Na^+ and K^+ along with water by infusion with 0.9%
(normal) saline with KCl supplementation. This would gradually
reverse the alkalosis with a rise in urinary pH over the ensuing
days.

Answer 3

(a) (i)   Surgical trauma stimulates anti-diuretic hormone pro-
          duction with retention of salt and water

2

    (ii) He would require no electrolyte supplements. Water
          requirements would be less than the normal daily re-
          quirement of 2–3 litres per day and would be determined
          by the CVP reading. Five per cent dextrose is transfused
          to keep the CVP at approximately 2–6 cm of water

2

(b) (i)   A normal CVP and BP would ensure good renal perfusion.
          A post-renal cause must be excluded by ensuring patency
          of catheter drainage. A low CVP is treated by volume
          replacement and a persistent low BP with pressure
          support using IV dopamine or dobutamine. The rate of
          elevation of serum urea and creatinine would indicate
          the extent of renal malfunction: this is nearly always due
          to acute tubular necrosis due to prolonged hypotension
          or a coagulopathy. A renal isotope scan would reveal the
          functional state of each kidney

4

(ii) Renal failure requires haemofiltration or haemodialysis to lower the urea and creatinine and to maintain electrolyte balance   2

Comment

Acute tubular necrosis is a sequela of major trauma, surgical or otherwise, where there is significant blood loss resulting in renal ischaemia. Cross-clamping the aorta in the vicinity of the renal arteries may also produce a fall in renal perfusion. Large volume transfusion with stored blood in the perioperative period may produce a coagulopathy, causing acute intravascular coagulation which may lead to renal damage and failure. Acute tubular necrosis usually recovers, and during recovery there is a diuresis, when large quantities of fluid and electrolytes are lost. Careful monitoring and replacement is therefore essential until complete renal function returns.

Answer 4

(a) (i) Pyrexial reactions are due to allergens and Gram-negative endotoxins in the donor blood. The skin rash is produced by agglutination of the donor cells due to incompatibility of the recipient serum and donor cells   2

(ii) Stop the transfusion immediately; set up a crystalloid infusion to produce a diuresis. Administer an antihistamine and an antipyretic agent as required   2

(b) (i) Acute liver failure and hepatic coma are rare complications and are precipitated by underlying liver disease. Some clotting factors are inactivated in stored blood, and a coagulopathy manifesting as acute intravascular coagulation leads to a bleeding diathesis in the postoperative period   2

(ii) In stored blood the plasma K^+ ions rise to 30–40 mmol/l and produce hyperkalaemia in the recipient. This may be treated by insulin administration with a covering dextrose infusion or by the ingestion of ion-exchange resin (calcium resonium). Citrated blood

	Marks
lowers the plasma Ca^{++} ion concentration in the recipient and it is treated by administration of calcium gluconate or calcium chloride	4

Comment

The signs of a mismatched blood transfusion include fever, chills, breathlessness, pain in the flanks and chest. These may be followed by hypotension, haemorrhagic phenomena and haemoglobinaemia. The last signals renal damage, which is exacerbated by hypotension and acidosis. The initial reactions occur during the first 30 minutes of the transfusion, and this period must be closely monitored when setting up a blood transfusion.

Answer 5

(a) (i)   Plastic apron and non-porous sterile gowns
      Visors or goggles
      Double gloving
      Theatre footwear with shoe covers   2

   (ii) Avoid passing instruments 'hand-to-hand'
      Avoid 'sharps' by using cutting diathermy instead of scalpel
      Scissors with bevelled ends
      Blunt needles
      Metal or plastic clips for haemostasis and wound closure   3

(b) (i)   Lowered platelet count
      Lowered vitamin K levels
      Raised prothrombin and partial thromboplastin times   2

   (ii) Lowered Hb
      Lowered WBC count
      Lowered serum albumin (hypoproteinaemia)
      Lowered immunoglobulins   3

Comment

The grave dangers of accidental inoculation with tissue fluids from HIV patients during operations should ensure familiarity with safety measures formulated to protect theatre personnel. Patients

with HIV infection have an increased risk of primary and   **Marks**
secondary haemorrhage and post-surgical bacterial infection.
Wound healing is also delayed due to hypoproteinaemia from
cachexia.

Answer 6

(a) (i)   Metabolic acidosis   1

    (ii) Ketoacidosis
        Lactic acidosis
        Renal failure   2

(b) (i)   Plasma glucose
        U&E and creatinine   3

    (ii) IV normal saline or Hartmann's solution
        IV K^+ infusion guided by U&E estimation
        IV insulin on a sliding scale
        IV antibiotics – flucloxacillin (or cefuroxime) and
        metronidazole
        Measure:
        4-hourly ABG
        4-hourly U&E
        2-hourly serum K^+ 4

Comment

A variety of organic acids are produced during metabolic activity
and their effects are counteracted by expelling CO_2 in the lungs
and excreting an acid urine. During metabolic or surgical illness
the body is unable to counter the acid load produced, leading to
metabolic acidosis. Determination of the base excess and HCO_3^-
in arterial blood enables effective countermeasures. In addition to
the measures stated, 4.8% $NaHCO_3$ IV infusion is indicated if the
acidosis is intractable or is causing cardiac arrhythmias, confu-
sion or drowsiness.

Answer 7

(a) (i)   He has been unable to eat or drink properly due to
        difficulty in swallowing   1

			Marks
	(ii)	Moderate to severe protein–calorie (energy) malnutrition	1
	(iii)	Visible muscle wasting with reduced muscle strength. Lax subcutaneous tissue from loss of fat deposits as shown by skinfold thickness	2
(b)	(i)	By enteral feeding through a fine-bore nasogastric tube or by total parenteral nutrition. By either route 1.5–2.5 litres of fluid containing 2000–2500 kcal and 1.5 g of protein per kg body weight is infused every 24 hours	3
	(ii)	Daily measurements of body weight Input and output fluid charts Serum U&Es, albumin, glucose and urinary glucose Twice-weekly measurements of Hb, Ca^{++}, Mg^{++}, triglycerides, urinary creatinine, Na^+ and K^+	3

Comment

Nutrient solutions, whether enteral or parenteral, must be administered in moderate increments during the first 48 hours to avoid hyperosmolarity of the body fluids and to give time for pancreatic adaptation. Extraneous insulin may be required to maintain the blood sugar within normal limits. Vitamins and trace elements are added daily. Skin callipers are used in some centres to quantify subcutaneous fat loss. A feeding gastrostomy or jejunostomy should be avoided if the patient is to undergo surgery for his stricture.

CHAPTER 2: TRAUMA AND BURNS

Answer 1   **Marks**

(a) Glasgow coma scale (see *Comment*)   2

(b) Blood pressure, pulse and respiration
     Pupillary sizes and reflexes
     Eye movements (extrinsic muscles)
     Abdominal reflexes; Cremasteric reflex
     Limbs: Tone
             Power, clonus
             Reflexes (triceps, biceps, brachioradialis, knee
             jerk, ankle jerk, plantar reflex)   3

(c) (i) Extra(epi)dural
          Subdural
          Subarachnoid
          Intracerebral
          CT/MRI Head scan   2

     (ii) Protect the airway
          Record blood pressure and pulse, with head injury
          observations ¼-hourly
          Daily arterial blood gases
          FBC and U&E
          Intracranial pressure monitoring
          Mannitol infusion preoperatively
          Surgical evacuation of haematoma
          Postoperative antibiotic therapy   3

Comment

Glasgow coma scale: Score

Eyes open { spontaneous   4/5
              to speech   3/4
              to pain   2
              none   1

				Marks
Verbal response	{	orientated	5	
		confused	4	
		inappropriate	3	
		incomprehensible	2	
		none	1	

Motor response	{	obeys commands	5
		localizes pain	4
		flexion to pain	3
		extension to pain	2
		none	1

Best total score   14/15

In all forms of intra-cranial bleeding, the time between injury and decompression is a major determinant of outcome. The onus should, therefore, be on rapid evacuation to a neurosurgical centre for appropriate management.

Recovery from intracranial haemorrhage is slow and unpredictable. The multidisciplinary rehabilitation team should include neurosurgical, psychiatric, speech and physiotherapy, and social and community services.

Answer 2

(a) Clinically assess airway patency and air exchange, viz oropharynx for foreign body or mucus plug obstruction, respiratory movements. Monitor pulse and BP. Establish peripheral and central venous access for CVP, ABG and pulmonary arterial wedge pressure measurements; FBC and U&E. Administer O_2 by face mask. Record ECG

3

(b) Tension/open pneumothorax (including flail chest)
Massive haemothorax
Cardiac tamponade

2

(c) (i) Promptly close defect in chest wall with sterile occlusive dressings large enough to overlap wound edges and tape securely on three sides to provide a flutter valve effect. Site a chest drain remote from the wound. Close the wound surgically when the patient's condition is stable

2

(ii) Decide drain site on CXR, usually at 5th intercostal space on anterior or mid-axillary line. Infiltrate area with lignocaine (1 or 2%) or bupivacaine (0.5%). Make skin incision, introduce tube drain on introducer into pleural cavity. Connect drain to under-water seal. Secure drain and close wound around it with non-absorbable sutures

Marks

3

Comment
Flail chest occurs when a segment of the chest wall becomes detached from the rib cage. It leads to 'paradoxical breathing' but may be initially masked due to splinting of the chest wall from pain. Mechanical ventilation is usually indicated.

Massive haemothorax results from a rapid loss of 1–2 litres of blood into the pleural cavity and must be suspected when shock is associated with absent breath sounds and dullness to percussion on that side. Initial management is by simultaneous restoration of blood volume and decompression of the pleural cavity. Continued blood loss (>200 ml/hr) may require thoracotomy.

Cardiac tamponade presents as paradoxical elevation of the JVP on inspiration, fall in arterial pulse pressure and muffled heart sounds (Beck's triad). Pericardiocentesis is indicated when response to resuscitation is poor and the diagnosis suspected. Tracings on a cardiac monitor may reveal injury patterns which along with a positive pericardiocentesis would require thoracotomy and inspection of the heart.

Answer 3

(a) (i) Right-sided tension pneumothorax
    Right haemothorax

2

   (ii) Tracheal shift to left
    Hyper-resonant or dull to percussion, with diminished or absent breath sounds in the right chest
    Evidence of injury to chest wall on gently springing the rib cage

2

	Marks
(b) (i) ABG	1

(ii) Postero-anterior and lateral chest X-ray   1

(c) Pulmonary contusion
Myocardial contusion
Aortic disruption
Diaphragmatic rupture
Tracheo-bronchial disruption
Oesophageal disruption   4

Comment

Pulmonary and myocardial contusions are the most common potentially lethal chest injuries. In the former, respiratory failure may be subtle and develop over time, and in the latter the diagnosis is made by abnormalities on the ECG. Traumatic aortic rupture is a cause of sudden death; potential survivors tend to have a laceration near the ligamentum anteriosum of the aorta, continuity being maintained by an intact adventitial layer. Many survivors die in hospital if the injury is unrecognised. A cardinal radiological sign is a widened mediastinum, caused by the haematoma surrounding the aorta. Blunt traumatic disruption to the tracheo-bronchial tree, oesophagus and diaphragm may all present late, and operative repair with drainage is life-saving. Unlike immediately life-threatening conditions these injuries may not be obvious on initial examination, and timely diagnosis is often based on a high index of clinical suspicion.

Answer 4

(a) (i) Liver, spleen, pancreas, duodenum, diaphragm, kidneys, urinary bladder   2

(ii) Ultrasound scan or CT of abdomen   1

(b) (i) Quarter-hourly BP, pulse and respiration
Check urine for blood
Half-hourly urine output; catheterize if required
FBC, ABG, CXR, AXR   2

		Marks

(ii) Peripheral and central venous access for volume re-placement and CVP monitoring. Intubation and me-chanical ventilation for respiratory decompensation 2

(c) Developing signs of peritonism and an increase in abdomi-nal girth signify intraperitoneal haemorrhage or rupture of a hollow viscus. Imaging of the abdomen or a diagnostic peritoneal lavage would detect bleeding and/or visceral injuries before the onset of lethal complications (oligaemia and/or toxic shock). 3

Comment

Unrecognised abdominal injury remains a frequent cause of preventable death after trauma. Peritoneal signs are often over-shadowed by pain from associated injuries. Diagnostic peritoneal lavage under local anaesthetic can alter subsequent physical signs but does reveal the presence of intraperitoneal bleeding or bowel contents. A laparoscopic examination under a general anaesthetic may be useful when a significant visceral injury is suspected. It will confirm the diagnosis and determine the extent of the injury that may require laparotomy.

Answer 5

(a) Resuscitation order:
Ensure airway patency and adequate ventilation by admin-istering supplementary oxygen
Restore circulatory blood volume by crystalloids, plasma expanders and colloids as necessary with pulse, BP and JVP monitoring
Alleviate pain with narcotic analgesics
Perform careful and thorough physical examination
Commence head injury observations and immobilise cervi-cal/dorsal spine if injury is suspected 5

(b) Counter hypothermia, administer O_2 by face mask, set up IV infusion and monitor vital signs
Maintain constant verbal and tactile communication and reassure the conscious patient
Treat life- and limb-threatening emergencies as facilities permit 3

(c) 1 anaesthetist
1 trauma surgeon
1 trauma nurse
1 paramedic
1 pilot
(Helicopter capacity rarely exceeds 6 persons, including the
patient and equipment)

2

Comment
Resuscitation is best carried out in the ambulance, except in
respiratory or cardiac arrest, when intubation and external cardiac
massage are performed at the roadside. When immediate extraction of the victim from the wreckage is not possible, life support is
continued and consideration given to the need for on-site amputation of a severely injured trapped limb.

Answer 6

(a) Cervical spine: fracture of vertebral arches or bodies with/
without dislocation. Cervical cord: concussion, incomplete
lesion, hemisection, transection

3

(b) Skin bruising on the lateral and/or posterior aspects of the
neck; neck muscle spasm

1

Attempt to elicit passive movement!

1

(c) (i) Reduction and stabilisation of fracture by cervical traction or internal fixation in selected patients

2

(ii) Care of nutritional requirements and prevention of cata-
bolic state
Prevention and treatment of respiratory and/or urinary
infections
Skin care to prevent pressure sores

3

Comment
Cervical spine injuries are caused by flexion, rotation, compression
and hyperextension. Indication for surgery is progression of neu-

rological deficit despite reduction and external stabilisation. **Marks**
Spinal fusion avoids prolonged bed rest with its associated
morbidity.

Answer 7

(a) (i) Use 'Rule of Nines' (modified for infants and toddlers)
Affected area: approximately 18%   1

    (ii) Verbal reassurance
Pain relief and sedation
Tetanus prophylaxis
Wound toilet: the burn surface is either left exposed or
covered with dressing impregnated with silver nitrate
or an antibiotic in an oil or water base
Prophylactic antibiotic therapy for 5–10 days   4

(b) (i) Partial thickness injury appears moist, red and blis-
tered, with preservation of pain sensation. Full-thickness injury is usually white or brown, dry, firm and   2
insensitive to touch

    (ii) Body weight in kg x % of burned surface = amount of
fluid in ml. This is the amount required in the first four
hours. Monitor haematocrit and hourly urine output
and give same amount over next four hours. Provided
the clinical state is stable, give the same amount over
the next 16 hours. (Approximately half colloid and half
crystalloid solutions)   3

Comment
The child may develop paralytic ileus and for the first 6–8 hours
the oral intake should be restricted to 50 ml of water per hour and
thereafter gradually increased to half-strength milk, followed by
a liquid diet.

Immediate tangential excision of the burn with split-skin grafting reduces fluid and protein loss, prevents infection and accel-
erates healing.

Answer 8 Marks

(a) Smoke inhalation injury (respiratory tract burns) 1

   Humidified oxygen by face mask
   Ambu-bag ventilation if required
   Calm patient with reassurance
   Mild sedation if necessary 2

(b) (i) Laryngeal oedema and/or oedema of the lower respiratory tract with bronchospasm 2

   (ii) Endotracheal intubation with assisted ventilation. Tracheostomy if prolonged mechanical ventilation is required 2

   (iii) Relieve bronchospasm with bronchodilators and steroids (as required). Positive pressure ventilation if arterial blood gases deteriorate. Prophylactic systemic antibiotic cover IV crystalloid administration to maintain hydration and renal function 3

Comment

Severe respiratory burns lead rapidly to respiratory failure and death. Lesser degrees of bronchial and alveolar damage lead to the 'shock lung syndrome', with increased airway resistance, raised pulmonary arterial wedge pressure and right ventricular strain. Continuous cardio-pulmonary support in an intensive therapy unit is required until lung function recovers.

Answer 9

(a) (i) Apply semi-rigid cervical collar
   Support spine during lifting and log rolling
   Strap patient in a neutral position on a back board for transfer to hospital with sand bags to support head, neck and shoulders 2

   (ii) A lateral X-ray showing the base of the skull, all seven cervical vertebrae and the first thoracic vertebra

An antero-posterior neck X-ray to include an open mouth odontoid view	**Marks**
An antero-posterior view of the dorsal spine	2

(b) (i) Flaccid areflexia, especially with a flaccid rectal sphincter
Diaphragmatic breathing
Passive flexion but not extension at the elbow
Grimaces to painful stimuli above but not below the clavicle
Hypotension with bradycardia
Priapism (an uncommon but characteristic sign)   3

(c) Neurogenic shock results from injury to descending sympathetic pathways in the spinal cord, with loss of vasomotor tone and sympathetic innervation to the heart. The former causes intravascular pooling of blood and consequent hypotension, and the latter causes inability to increase the heart rate and produces bradycardia. The blood pressure, therefore, cannot be restored by fluid infusion alone, and the judicious use of vasopressor agents may be required   3

Comment
Three tracts are readily assessed clinically in evaluating a spinal cord injury. The corticospinal tract controls motor power on the same side and is tested by voluntary muscle contractions or involuntary response to painful stimuli. The spinothalamic tract transmits pain and temperature sensations to the opposite side and is tested by pinch or pin prick. The posterior columns carry proprioceptive impulses from the same side and are tested by position sense of the fingers and toes or tuning fork vibrations. A complete spinal cord lesion abolishes distal neurological function and prognosis for recovery is poor. Incomplete spinal cord lesions are compatible with recovery, and a careful examination to determine the presence of any sensory or motor function is, therefore, essential.

Answer 10

(a) (i) Primary survey detects tracheal deviation and rib injury (by gently springing the rib cage) and the presence of: **Marks**

    Central cyanosis
    Paradoxical breathing
    Surgical emphysema
    Abdominal skin bruising or tenderness   2

(ii) AXR, ultrasound scan and/or CT of abdomen and pelvis and/or diagnostic peritoneal lavage or laparoscopic examination
Catheterize and examine urine for blood   2

(iii) Gentle palpation for a fracture and/or dislocation
Antero-posterior and lateral X-rays of the hip, femur, knee, tibia, fibula and ankle   2

(b) Establish two large-calibre IV peripheral lines
Establish a central venous line for CVP monitoring
Send blood for FBC, ABG, grouping and emergency cross-match
Transfuse with crystalloid solution (e.g. Ringer lactate) and a plasma volume expander (e.g. Haemacel) until whole blood is available to restore blood volume   4

Comment

The pulse and BP are monitored quarter-hourly, though these are poor measures of tissue perfusion. A pulse oximeter measures the saturation of haemoglobin colorimetrically (it is not a measure of partial pressure of oxygen). A small sensor is clipped onto the finger, toe or earlobe and displays the pulse rate and oxygen concentration continuously and reflects the respiratory and circulatory status.

Hypovolaemic shock should not be treated with fluid replacement alone. Once the circulatory blood volume has been replaced and if tissue perfusion has not recovered due to peripheral vascular shutdown, judicious use of steroids and pressor agents to maintain renal and cerebral perfusion may be appropriate in an intensive care setting.

Answer 11

(a) Extent: Chest and abdomen make up 18% and each arm 7% of total body surface area ('Rule of Nines' modified for infants and toddlers)

Depth: Partial-thickness or epidermal scald blanches on pressure, is pink and may blister, and is painful with a positive pinprick. Full-thickness scald does not blanch, is pale or dull brown, and is devoid of pain (negative pinprick)   3

(b) Scalds exceeding 10% of body surface or a full-thickness scald exceeding 2.5cm²

Unrelated but significant underlying illness, e.g. diabetes, heart disease or epilepsy

Injury suspected of being non-accidental

Poor home circumstances   3

(c) Open method: Expose surface moistened with antibacterial agents, in an environment of sterile ambient air, or Closed method: Cover area with sterile occlusive non-adherent dressings impregnated with antibacterial agents. These are: Chlorhexidine-impregnated tulle gras, has anti-staphylococcal action; 1% sulphadiazine cream, has anti Gram-negative action (e.g. *Pseudomonas*, *Klebsiella*, *E. coli*); 10% Sulphamylon cream, has same spectrum as above but penetrates avascular tissue; 0.5% silver nitrate solution soaked in cotton gauze, is bacteriostatic   4

Comment

Details of the circumstances of the injury must be obtained from an accompanying adult. The temperature of the liquid, whether clothing was worn, the exposure time, and if the surface was cooled with tap water or cold milk soon afterwards, are important in assessing wound depth and prognosis. The time interval between scalding and presentation, if more than six hours, is likely to result in an infection. Tetanus prophylaxis or immunisation is administered on presentation; pain relief, sedation and oral intake following IV hydration is monitored in the ensuing days. Bacterial colonization of the injured surface is usually

complete in 24–48 hours. This may manifest as a local infection **Marks**
or may result in systemic spread, with fever and rigors. Prophylactic antibiotic therapy is therefore indicated in scalds exceeding
10% of the surface.

Answer 12

(a) Level of consciousness: GCS score chart
     Airway patency and respiratory function
     Cardiac function by recording the pulse, BP and electrical
     activity on a cardiac monitor   3

(b) Full-thickness burn wounds at entry and exit sites with
     variable underlying tissue destruction and damage to inter-
     vening tissue, viz subcutaneous fat and muscle   3

(c) Heart: ectopic rhythms, arrhythmias, ventricular fibrillation
     leading to cardiac arrest
     Kidneys: acute renal failure due to (i) reduced perfusion
     during the shock phase, (ii) released haemoglobin red cells
     and damaged muscle
     Muscle: tetanic contractions leading to joint and soft tissue
     injuries
     Brain: convulsions leading to cerebral oedema
     Peripheral nerves: conduction defects   4

Comment
Immediate cardiopulmonary resuscitation is commenced in ventricular arrhythmias. ECG monitoring and cardiac enzyme estimations detect injury to the heart muscle. Tissue destruction in high voltage electrical injuries is extensive and may progress as initially viable tissue necroses, due to vascular thrombosis and capillary damage. In addition to wound debridement, excision of dead or poorly viable muscle is required to prevent myoglobinuria and gas gangrene. Wounds must be left open, as progressive muscle necrosis is likely and may require further debridement. Early fasciotomy may be required if limb swelling progresses, to preserve its blood supply.

Answer 13

(a) The loss of serous fluid from the burned surface is replaced
     by plasma in the form of plasma protein fraction (PPF) or
     fresh frozen plasma (FFP) in four-hourly alliquots calcu-
     lated as follows:

$$\% \text{ burn area x patient's body weight x } \tfrac{1}{2} \text{ (in ml)}$$

This initial guide is influenced by the clinical, haematological
and biochemical profiles during the 24-hour period   3

(b) Wound debridement and toilet
     Keep wound surface warm and moist with open or closed
     methods
     Take wound culture swabs from multiple sites daily
     Cover burned area early by homografts or heterografts
     which are renewed in the ward until the entire area is
     autografted from the patient's own donor sites
     Correct dehydration, hypoproteinaemia and anaemia
     Ensure adequate oral nutritional intake   4

(c) Ensure adequate pain relief with IV opiates and optimal
     fluid and electrolyte balance
     The patient may only have a few hours of clarity of thought
     left before lapsing into confusion or coma. Therefore, ex-
     plain the probable outcome and prognosis and the therapeu-
     tic options gently and dispassionately so that the patient's
     wishes on further management may be adhered to. Maxim-
     ise time spent with loved ones and relatives with ready
     access to counsellor or priest. Seclude the patient from
     extraneous ward activity.   3

Comment

The extent of the burn injury is estimated by the 'Rule of Nines'.
The depth of the burn should be mapped out and may be broadly
divided into superficial (partial thickness) or deep (full thickness). The former involves the epidermis and superficial layers of
the dermis and, in the latter, the epidermis and dermis are
destroyed with a variable extent of underlying tissue. A third type

that is occasionally seen is the deep dermal burn where some of the germinal layers are spared but healing is poor and protracted, with wound contracture and scarring. Flame burns are nearly always deep, and the burn surface is debrided by tangential excision and covered by 'split skin' grafts taken from the patient's own donor sites. However, when the burn area is larger than the available donor sites, banked cadaver or pig skin may be used as temporary dressings until the area is grafted in stages by the patient's own skin. The former must be renewed every few days to prevent adherence and bleeding. There is no reliable evidence that using such 'other skin' dressings is superior to conventional antiseptic-impregnated, non-adherent gauze. Survival following a burn injury is dependent on the patient's age, the burn area and depth. In the very young, the very old and the chronically ill, the morbidity is high, from complications of the burn injury.

Answer 1

Marks

(a) Muscle spasm resulting in restricted range of movements, namely of abduction and internal rotation. A soft tissue swelling may be present

3

(b) (i) Perthes' disease (osteochondritis of the femoral epiphysis): collapse/fragmentation of ossification centre resulting in flattening of femoral head

(ii) Slipped upper femoral epiphysis: displacement of femoral epiphysis

(iii) Tuberculosis of the hip. Loss of bone density adjacent to joint with narrowing of joint space; later bone destruction, with abscess formation

4

(c) In Perthes' disease and slipped epiphysis, avascular necrosis leads to progressive deformity and osteoarthritis in early adult life

In tuberculosis, complete destruction of the joint, with abscess and later sinus formation; systemic spread may lead to a fatal outcome

3

Comment
The pathogenesis of Perthes' disease and slipped upper femoral epiphysis is ischaemia of the femoral head. Both occur between the ages of 5–15 years, when the femoral head depends on the lateral epiphyseal vessels for its blood supply. Tuberculosis of the hip joint is usually secondary to primary disease in the lung or the bowel and is accompanied by constitutional symptoms. A chest X-ray and a positive Mantoux test are required to support the diagnosis.

Answer 2

(a) Injury is dependent on the extent of rotation and is progressive as follows: Tear of anterior part of lateral ligament leads to fractures of lateral malleolus and then medial malleolus (bimalleolar fracture). Tear of the medial ligament leads to fracture of posterior articular surface of tibia which may extend to a trimalleolar fracture dislocation (Pott's fracture)

Marks

4

(b) Proximal fibular fracture with diastasis of the inferior tibio-fibular joint and disruption of the interosseous tibio-fibular ligament

2

(c) Principle: restoration of normal ankle mortice
Unstable ankle fractures may be treated with

- external reduction and immobilization in above-knee plaster cast; weightbearing is avoided for 4–6 weeks

- internal fixation: (this prevents late displacement) and early mobilization

4

Comment
One of the most common diagnostic errors in ankle injuries is to miss a proximal fibular fracture; X-rays must include the knee and ankle joints. Failure of effective treatment of ankle diastasis leads to permanent ankle instability.

Answer 3

(a) (i) Rheumatoid arthritis

1

   (ii) Stage 1 – synovitis: thickening of capsule, villous formation of synovium and a cell rich effusion into the joint and tendon sheaths
   Stage 2 – destruction: articular cartilage, and tendon sheaths are eroded
   Stage 3 – deformity: the combination of articular destruction, capsular stretching and tendon rupture leads to progressive instability and deformity of the joint

3

(b) Normocytic, hypochromic anaemia
Rise in ESR, C reactive protein and oncoproteins
Rheumatoid factor present in 80% and antinuclear factor in 30% of patients

3

(c) Stop synovitis, prevent deformity, reconstruct the joint and   **Marks**
     rehabilitate the patient, using a multidisciplinary approach   3

Comment
There is no cure for rheumatoid arthritis. Joint pain and swelling
due to the synovitis is reduced by bed rest and non-steroidal anti-
inflammatory agents. Systemic corticosteroids give effective relief
of symptoms but have serious side effects. Intra-synovial injec-
tions of corticosteroids and cytotoxic drugs reduce joint inflammation, as do systemically administered gold, penicillamine,
hydroxychloroquine and methotrexate (immunosuppression). Joint
splinting, physiotherapy and postural training may prevent progressive deformity. Deformity associated with loss of function and
pain is treated by joint reconstruction or joint replacement.

Answer 4

(a) Decreased joint space due to thinning of cartilage
     Subarticular sclerosis
     Subchondral cyst formation
     Osteophyte formation   3

(b) Analgesics and warmth
     Non-steroidal anti-inflammatory agents
     Preservation of movement by non-weightbearing exercises
     Adjustment of activities to reduce stress on the hip   3

(c) (i)   Progressive increase in pain
           Severe restriction of activities
           Marked deformity
           Progressive loss of movement, in particular abduction
           Radiological signs of joint destruction   3

     (ii) Total hip replacement   1

Comment
Primary osteoarthritis is common in the fifth and sixth decades of
life and has no apparent underlying cause. The articular cartilage
becomes soft and fibrillated, and the underlying bone shows cyst
formation and sclerosis. Synovial hypertrophy and capsular fibrosis cause joint stiffness. Re-alignment osteotomy may arrest or

slow further cartilage destruction, whilst arthrodesis of the hip **Marks**
produces freedom from pain and stability, at the expense of
mobility. Total replacement arthroplasty using a prosthesis replacing the acetabulum as well as the head of the femur is the
operation of choice.

Answer 5

(a) Closed reduction under general anaesthetic with longitudi-
     nal traction on forearm, gradually flexing the elbow
     Correct lateral displacement during traction
     Monitor radial pulse throughout
     Apply a back slab to flexed elbow, and a collar and cuff
     Admit overnight to monitor limb circulation
     Immobilize for three weeks   4

(b) Ischaemia of forearm and hand due to arterial injury, arterial
     spasm or swelling of flexor compartment
     Treatment: remove all dressings; reduce fracture immedi-
     ately
     Do not overflex a badly swollen arm
     If the radial pulse does not return, surgical decompression
     of the forearm and/or exploration of the brachial artery at the
     vicinity of the fracture   3

(c) Injury to brachial artery/vein
     Injury to nerves
     Epiphyseal damage
     Stiffness and delayed functional recovery
     Volkmann's ischaemic contracture   3

Comment

The importance of this fracture is the associated neuro-vascular
injury. Monitoring the radial pulse during and immediately after
reduction is of cardinal importance in avoiding ischaemic injury.
Pulse, hand sensation and finger movements must be monitored,
preferably overnight, to detect possible nerve or vessel compression. If closed reduction is not possible without compromising the
brachial artery, open reduction or Dunlop traction (longitudinal
traction via a pin in the olecranon) may be used.

Answer 6   **Marks**

(a) The condition must be looked for during routine exami-
    nation
    Abduct both hips with knees and hips flexed to a right angle
    – the 'click' of reduction of a subluxated/dislocated hip is
    diagnostic
    Subluxated hips are reduced and maintained in abduction
    with double nappies
    Dislocated hips are reduced and held in an abduction splint
    (frog plaster spica)   5

(b) Joint laxity due to unfavourable intrauterine posture, or
    genetic or placental hormonal factors
    Dysplasia of the hip with deficient acetabulum and/or femo-
    ral head   2

(c) Treatment of established condition is difficult due to adap-
    tive changes
    Reduction of hip by closed or open method and maintained
    for at least six weeks
    Any residual deformity is corrected by osteotomy. Acetabular
    dysplasia may require surgical correction at a later stage   3

Comment
Subluxated hips are not uncommon at birth (5–10 per 1000). Most
reduce spontaneously soon after birth. Failure to diagnose and
correct the dislocation before the child starts walking is negligent,
as a good result is then difficult to achieve; osteoarthritis is a likely
late complication.

Answer 7

(a) (i) Acute osteomyelitis of the radius/ulna   1

    (ii) Aspirate from area of maximal inflammation and send
         fluid for Gram staining and culture to identify the
         causative organism and its sensitivity
         Raised WBC, ESR and anti-staphylococcal antibody
         titres   3

(b)   Cellulitis of the forearm   **Marks**
      Acute suppurative arthritis of elbow
      Sickle cell crisis
      Gaucher's disease (pseudo-osteitis)   3

(c)   Analgesia and rehydration
      Splint the forearm
      Antibiotic therapy; initially broad spectrum, later sensitivity
      specific
      Surgical drainage if abscess has formed   3

Comment

Plain X-rays are of limited value during the first few days, as there is little or no radiological abnormality of the bone. By the end of the second week, periosteal new bone formation and metaphyseal mottling may be present – the classic X-ray signs of pyogenic osteomyelitis: treatment should never be delayed while waiting for these signs to appear. Cellulitis of the forearm may present an identical clinical picture and, in tropical climates, pyomyositis (inflammation of skeletal muscle) is caused by the same organisms. Accompanying septicaemia and fever may cause severe dehydration, and intravenous fluids may be required.

Answer 8

(a)   (i)   Childhood rickets   1

      (ii)   X-rays: thickening and widening of epiphysis, cupping
           of the metaphysis, bowing of diaphysis   2

      (iii) Biochemistry: reduced serum Ca^{++} and PO_4^{---}
           ($Ca \times PO_4 < 2.4$ diagnostic)
           Raised serum alkaline phosphatase   2

(b)   (i)   Underexposure to sunlight
           Vitamin D deficiency from poor diet (or post-gastrectomy
           in adults) or malabsorption due to coeliac or pancreatic
           disease or small bowel surgery
           Chronic liver or kidney disease   3

(ii) Dietary vitamin D supplementation with α-calcidol (vitamin D analogue) or calciferol (vitamin D_2) up to 40,000 units daily — 2

Comment

In children bowing of the tibia if marked may require the wearing of callipers to prevent further deformity and to restore normal alignment until new bone formation occurs.

In adults the deficiency manifests as osteomalacia. The bones become deformed with an accompanying muscle weakness; correction of the deformities is by osteotomy.

Answer 9

(a) (i) Paget's disease of the spine (osteitis deformans) — 1

(ii) Areas of osteoclastic activity with bone reabsorption, giving a radiological flame-shaped lesion externally along the shaft of bone
Adjacent areas of osteoblastic activity, with new bone formation, leading to radiological sclerosis and coarse trabeculation
Fibrovascular tissue is laid down in areas of bone excavation — 4

(b) Spinal stenosis with nerve root compression
Pathological fracture
Osteoarthritis
Bone sarcoma — 2

(c) Non-steroidal anti-inflammatory agents for bone and joint pain. Suppression of bone turnover by calcitonin and diphosphorates – effective when the disease is in active phase
Calcitonin decreases osteoclastic activity
Diphosphorates reduce bone growth by binding to hydroxyapatite crystals — 3

Comment

Most people with Paget's disease are asymptomatic, and the

disease comes to light during X-ray investigation for an unre-   **Marks**
lated condition. Surgery is reserved for complications of pathological fractures (internal fixation with straightening of the
bone) and for nerve entrapment due to severe spinal stenosis
(surgical decompression). Osteogenic sarcoma, if detected early,
may be resectable. A high output cardiac failure and
hypercalcaemia may also be associated with the disease.

Answer 10

(a) (i) Tuberculosis of the dorsal spine (Pott's disease of the
         spine)   1

    (ii) Destruction of adjacent vertebral bodies by caseation
         leads to collapse, producing spinal angulation. The
         paravertebral abscess tracks down deep to the psoas
         fascia and points in the groin   2

(b) Mantoux/Heaf skin test – positive
    Raised ESR
    Plain chest X-ray – evidence of primary lung lesion
    X-ray of entire spine – to detect distant occult lesions and to
    assess the degree of angulation and the number of vertebrae
    and disc spaces involved at the kyphosis
    CT or MRI scan for evidence of impending cord compression
    Needle aspiration of the groin abscess for histological and
    bacteriological confirmation   3

(c) (i) Eradicate the disease with anti-tuberculous chemo-
         therapy
         Correct deformity and prevent spinal complications by
         drainage of paravertebral abscess and evacuation of
         infected/necrotic material
         Correction of angulation with strut (rib) grafts and
         spinal fusion
         Physiotherapy of the affected joints. High protein diet   3

    (ii) Pott's paraplegia   1

Comment   **Marks**

There is usually a long history of poor health and backache. Occasionally the patient may present with paraesthesia and weakness of the legs. Spinal tuberculosis should be distinguished from other causes of vertebral destruction, i.e. pyogenic infections and malignant disease. Tumour metastases may cause vertebral body collapse but, in contrast to tuberculous spondylitis, the disc space is usually preserved.

Answer 11

(a) (i) Acute osteomyelitis of radius/ulna
         Acute pyomyositis of flexor/extensor muscles   2

    (ii) The forearm is held still across the chest with the elbow
         flexed
         Elbow and wrist movements are present, though the
         range of movements is restricted due to muscle spasm or
         bone pain   2

(b) (i) *Staphylococcus aureus*
         Streptococcus pyogenes
         Haemophilus influenzae
         Pneumococcus
         Salmonella   2

    (ii) Acute osteomyelitis and pyomyositis in the early phase
         respond well to antibiotic therapy
         Sensitivity-specific agents are used once the organisms
         are isolated
         Generally, however, IV cloxacillin 200 mg/kg daily in
         divided doses – followed once the infection is under
         control by oral flucloxacillin 100 mg daily
         In penicillin allergies, a cephalosporin or fusidic acid
         and erythromycin may be substituted
         Malnutrition must be treated with urgent dietary meas-
         ures
         No surgical measures are required in the early acute
         phase of either illness

Abscess formation requires drainage, and bone necrosis   **Marks**
may occur in chronic osteomyelitis with involucrum
formation, when surgical debridement is required   4

Comment
The aetiology of myositis and osteomyelitis is associated with a
multitude of predisposing factors. Systemic bacterial infections,
e.g. staphylococcal bacteraemia may lead to seeding of the blood-
borne organism in damaged or ischaemic muscle or bone. The
presence of avitaminosis and malnutrition has led to dietary
factors, and chronic bowel infections with an overgrowth of
intestinal organisms being linked with muscle and bone infections in these children.

CHAPTER 4: NEUROSURGERY

Answer 1 Marks

(a) (i) Infantile hydrocephalus 1

  (ii) Tense anterior fontanelle
  'Cracked pot' sound on percussion
  Transillumination of cranial cavity
  'Setting sun' appearance of the eyes
  Thin scalp with dilated veins
  Abnormally large skull compared with normal growth
  charts 3

  (iii) CT or MRI head scan 1

(b) (i) Stenosis of aqueduct of Sylvius causes a sustained rise in
  intracranial pressure

  (ii) Spina bifida
  Meningomyelocele 2

(c) Cerebrospinal fluid shunt with a one-way valve between the
  lateral ventricle and right atrium or peritoneum 3

Comment
Hydrocephalus may be diagnosed prenatally by ultrasonography.
Treatment of infantile hydrocephalus is by shunting, except in the
rare chronic (arrested) hydrocephalus, where the cerebrospinal
fluid pressure has returned to normal. These children require
careful neurological follow-up to detect any deterioration. Following shunting, ventricular size can be monitored by ultrasonography
through the open anterior fontanelle. The overall prognosis is
poor, with one-third dying and one-third achieving a semblance of
normality by the age of 10 years.

Answer 2

(a) (i) Intracranial space-occupying lesion 1

  (ii) Raised intracranial pressure due to tumour mass with or
  without obstruction of cerebrospinal fluid circulation

Fits may be due to mass effect or pressure on motor pathways		**Marks** 3

(b) (i) Cranial CT or MRI scan
        Cerebral angiography   2

    (ii) Herniation of the brain stem into the foramen magnum   1

(c) Benign tumours:
        Meningioma
        Acoustic neuroma
        Haemangioblastoma
        Epidermoid and dermoid cysts
        Colloid cyst of the third ventricle
    Malignant tumours:
        Neuroepithelial tumour
        Germ cell tumour
        Lymphomas and leukaemias
        Metastatic tumours   3

Comment

Epilepsy is the most frequent initial symptom of a glioma or meningioma. Headaches that are present on waking, on changing posture, coughing, straining or of unusual intensity, and occurring in those not previously prone to headaches merit CT scanning. Changes in personality, cognitive function and memory are also features suggestive of brain tumour.

Answer 3

(a) (i) Subarachnoid haemorrhage due to ruptured cerebral aneurysm or arterio-venous malformation   2

    (ii) Increasing drowsiness leading to stupor and coma simultaneously mild focal neurological deficit may progress to moderate and then severe hemiparesis leading to decerebrate rigidity   3

(b) (i) CT or MRI head scan   1

	Marks
(ii) Xanthochromia and sterile CSF	1

(c) Medical measures:
    Bed rest, sedation and adequate analgesia
    Treat hypertension when present
    Maintain fluid and electrolyte balance
  Surgery:
    Control bleeding by clipping the aneurysm or feeding
    vessels to arterio-venous malformation   3

Comment

A sudden bleed into the subarachnoid space is soon followed by cerebral oedema and a raised intra-cranial pressure. Lumbar puncture in these circumstances may cause coning. If, however, fulminant meningitis cannot be ruled out, it may be carried out once the intra-cranial pressure stabilizes. Nimodipine, a calcium channel blocker, reduces the incidence of infarction and ischaemic deficits when administered soon after the haemorrhage.

Answer 4

(a) (i) Right hemiparesis/hemiplegia
     Dysphasia
     Right-sided sensory disturbance   2

   (ii) Hypertension; polycythaemia; diabetes mellitus; alcoholism; smoking; hyperlipidaemia
     Atrial fibrillation or valvular heart disease   2

(b) Cranial CT or MRI scan to evaluate the extent of cerebral infarction and oedema, and presence of intra-cranial haemorrhage
Maintain airway
Anticoagulation with IV heparin 40,000 units/24 hours if cause is embolic/thrombotic
Lower raised intra-cranial pressure: positive pressure ventilation with 5% PCO_2
Reduce cerebral oedema: Mannitol infusion and/or corticosteroid therapy
Maintain fluid, electrolyte and acid–base balance   6

Comment

Investigations should be directed towards categorizing the vascular event as a guide to prognosis. Surgical measures for improving cerebral perfusion or for cerebral decompression do not generally improve prognosis. Surgery may have a role in preventing subsequent stroke in those who survive the initial event.

Answer 5

(a) A history of a prodromal period with malaise, fever and listlessness
Clinical features of an underlying source of infection
Focal neurological signs (including epileptic fits)
Change in level of consciousness, i.e. drowsiness or irritability   3

(b) (i)   Streptococcus
Staphylococcus aureus
Proteus
Bacteroides fragilis
Escherichia coli
Haemophilus influenzae   2

(ii) Bronchitis/pneumonia
Otitis media
Sinus infection
Gastroenteritis   2

(c) Correct fluid and electrolyte balance
Sedation
Initially broad spectrum antimicrobial therapy then specific agent(s) once pus culture and sensitivity are available
Surgical aspiration or excision   3

Comment

A brain abscess is a mass lesion producing focal neurological signs and must be distinguished from meningitis. Lumbar puncture is contraindicated due to the danger of tentorial herniation.

Antibiotic therapy: the initial choice of antibiotic before culture results are available will depend on the probable cause of the abscess and the Gram stain.

Aspiration of an abscess may be performed by use of CT-guided stereotaxis. Aspiration may need to be repeated with CT follow-up. Surgical excision is indicated:

- For persistent re-accumulation despite repeated aspirations
- If the abscess is not accessible for aspiration
- In the presence of a fibrous capsule surrounding the abscess preventing collapse on aspiration

Answer 6

(a) Cervical cord lesion causing compression: extradural abscess; metastatic tumours; intradural tumours, e.g. meningioma, Schwannoma; intramedullary tumours, e.g. gliomas

Spinal lesions causing compression: cervical spondylolisthesis/spondylitis; intervertebral disc prolapse; infections of vertebral body (e.g. Pott's disease)   3

(b) Muscle wasting and lower motor neurone weakness, with sensory disturbance of nerve roots C5 to T1   3

(c) (i) Plain cervical spine X-rays
Myelography
CT scan (with intrathecal contrast) or MRI   2

(ii) Mild symptoms due to degenerative lesions of the spine respond well to analgesics, rest, physiotherapy and wearing of a collar
Surgical decompression of the cervical cord is required occasionally as an emergency for progressive neurological signs
Radiotherapy with corticosteroids is indicated for malignant cord compression   2

Comment

A feature of spinal cord compression is local and radicular pain which predates sensory and motor disturbances. Urinary sphincter disturbances may also be present. The tingling, or 'electric shock' sensation on flexion/extension of the neck (Lhemitte's sign) is diagnostic. Metastatic tumour deposits are from the lung, breast, kidney and prostate. Tumours of the reticulo-endothelial system also metastasise to the spine. Urgent surgery is required for progressive neurological signs to avoid permanent disability. Local palliative radiotherapy in malignant disease relieves pain and may produce a partial remission of weakness. It may be as effective in metastatic disease as surgical decompression.

Answer 1

(a) Occlusion of central retinal artery or vein
Ischaemic optic neuropathy
Retinal detachment
Vitreous haemorrhage
Temporal arteritis
Hysterical blindness
Macular lesions   4

(b) Atherosclerosis
Hypertension
Diabetes mellitus   3

(c) Any lesion involving the optic chiasma, including ischaemic
infarction
Hysterical blindness   3

Comment

The fundus in central retinal artery occlusion is creamy white due
to an infarcted retina, except over the macula, which is visible as
'the cherry red spot'. In ischaemic optic neuropathy (due to
temporal arteritis), a pale and swollen optic disc is present; in
retinal detachment the opaque retina obscures the normal choroidal
red glow, and instead there is a grey, rippling reflex.

Answer 2

(a) Conjunctivitis
Episcleritis and scleritis
Keratitis
Uveitis   2

(b) Look for a foreign body in the conjunctiva
Pupillary reflexes to light
Slit lamp examination of iris and lens
Fundoscopic examination of the retina
Fluorescein stain for corneal abrasions/ulcer   4

(c)	Retinoblastoma:	**Marks**
	Enucleation with chemo and/or radiotherapy	4

Comment
Red eye in the adult: three major causes are iritis, keratitis and acute angle closure (acute glaucoma). Signs on slit lamp examination are ciliary injection and white deposits on the corneal surface in iritis; a broken corneal epithelium in keratitis; and a hazy cornea with a shallow anterior chamber and a dilated pupil in acute glaucoma.

Answer 3

(a) (i) Acute orbital cellulitis   1

   (ii) Conjunctival and nasopharyngeal swabs for culture and sensitivity
Aerobic and anaerobic blood cultures

       AP and lateral X-rays of paranasal sinuses and orbit   2

(b) (i) Broad spectrum IV antibiotic therapy changing if required to sensitivity-specific
IV rehydration
Pain relief and sedation as required   2

   (ii) Place on a pulse and temperature chart
Test visual acuity and pupillary reaction twice daily and examine the optic disc daily
Serial ultrasound or CT scan to detect early signs of subperiosteal abscess formation   2

(c) (i) Surgical drainage and/or excision of the ethmoidal sinus, with drainage of frontal and sphenoidal sinuses   2

   (ii) Cavernous sinus thrombosis, which may lead to a brain abscess   1

Comment
Acute orbital cellulitis is the most common cause of exophthalmos in children and usually spreads from an infected ethmoid sinus.

Preseptal cellulitis, which is a common complication of acute sinusitis, may spread to the orbit, as orbital septa are not well developed in children. Following recovery on antibiotic therapy, the underlying paranasal sinusitis must be treated to prevent recurrences. Orbital surgical exploration is required if the infection cannot be controlled by antibiotics, with the danger of the infection spreading to the globe (panophthalmitis).

Marks

Answer 4

(a) (i) Blow-out fracture of the orbital floor   1

(ii) A hard object larger than 5 cm in diameter striking the orbit causes a sudden increase in intraorbital pressure, which produces orbital floor fracture   2

(b) (i) Infraorbital nerve injury causes anaesthesia involving the lower eyelid, cheek, side of nose, upper lip and teeth. Diplopia, when present, is typically vertical in both up-and-down gaze and is caused by tethering of extra-ocular muscles to the fracture line. Enophthalmos may be present initially or may appear later as the periorbital oedema subsides and the eyeball sinks into the fractured floor   3

(ii) Plain orbital X-rays (Waters' view)
CT scan of orbit (axial and coronal sections)   1

(c) Small cracks in the orbital floor without diplopia require no treatment. Fractures of less than 50% of the floor, with improving diplopia, require no treatment unless enophthalmos is more than 2 mm. Fractures of over 50% of the floor, with persistent diplopia, should be repaired within two weeks of injury   3

Comment
Despite the invariable presence of conjunctival ecchymosis and chemosis, orbital injuries rarely cause ocular damage. Surgical treatment of orbital floor fractures entails freeing the entrapped tissue and covering the defect with a plastic plate. Orbital margins

offer little protection to smaller missiles, such as squash balls and shuttlecocks that may impact directly onto the eyeball and cause serious ocular injury.

Marks

Answer 5

(a) Chronic laryngitis due to vocal abuse, tobacco use or myxoedema
Laryngeal polyps, nodules, granulomas and papillomas

2

(b) Indirect laryngoscopy by use of a laryngeal mirror with or without pharyngeal anaesthetic spray
Fibreoptic laryngoscopy via nostril with topical anaesthetic spray
Direct laryngoscopy under general anaesthetic (e.g. in children)

4

(c) Radiotherapy for most early lesions – with a cure rate of 90%
Laser beam surgical excision of early lesions is also curative
For extensive cord carcinomas, a partial or total laryngectomy may be performed in conjunction with a neck dissection for nodal involvement
Total laryngectomy requires a tracheostomy and oesophageal voice training

4

Comment
Laryngeal nodules, a specific and localized form of chronic laryngitis, are found in professional voice users (singer's nodules) and in children (screamer's nodules). Juvenile papillomas must be excluded in hoarseness in children; they are due to the human papilloma virus.

Carcinomas may present above (supra-glottic) or below (infra-glottic) the vocal cords. They have a worse prognosis than glottic tumours, as hoarseness is a late symptom and diagnosis being delayed until the cord is involved; the greater vascularity and lymphatic drainage above and below the cord predisposes to earlier metastases.

Answer 6 **Marks**

(a) (i) Conductive deafness caused by secretory otitis media is
        due to Eustachian tube dysfunction   2

  (ii) Predisposition:
        Acute otitis media
        Adenoidal inflammation
        Post-nasal space neoplasm
        Barotrauma   2

(b) There is reduced mobility of the eardrum, with hyperaemia
    The middle ear effusion may alter in composition and appear
    golden-brown or blue
    Occasionally bubbles may be seen through the drum
    A retracted drum with prominent malleus and occasional
    vesicles   2

(c) Myringotomy: aspiration of fluid under a general anaesthetic
    if troublesome symptoms persist for over three months

    Insertion of a grommet (a tiny flanged Teflon tube) into the
    drum is frequently required to avoid recurrence of middle ear
    fluid
    An anterior or inferior radial myringotomy incision is used to
    insert the grommet   4

Comment

Secretory otitis media may settle spontaneously. Nasal vasoconstrictor drops with an oral decongestant may assist recovery when there is an associated upper respiratory tract infection.

A marked and persistent hearing loss interfering with schooling necessitates surgery. This may involve the insertion of a grommet to drain and ventilate the middle ear. The grommet usually extrudes spontaneously 6–18 months after insertion. If normal Eustachian tube function has not returned and secretory otitis media recurs, the grommet is replaced.

Answer 7   Marks

(a) (i)   The lesion: the edge, base, floor and surrounding skin
          Regional lymph nodes   1

  (ii) Malignant melanoma   1

  (iii) Depth of invasion is measured from the top of the
        granular layer of the epidermis to the deepest melanoma
        cell in the dermis
        Tumour thickness < 0.76 mm has a favourable progno-
        sis   2

(b) Wide local excision down to deep fascia
     If histologically malignant:
     Radiotherapy with/without nodal clearance and/or chemo-
     therapy based on histological staging   3

(c) Protection from sun by clothing and wide-brimmed hats
     Apply sun screen lotions containing skin protection factors
     and limit time of exposure   3

Comment
Malignant change in a pre-existing naevus is difficult to assess as
there is uncertainty whether melanomas always arise from
pigmented moles. However, a change in size, itchiness or bleeding should arouse suspicion. Delayed or missed diagnosis may
result in dissemination, though it is unclear if this occurs during
the radial or vertical growth phases. Diagnosis is by histological
examination of the whole lesion, and incisional biopsy is, therefore, deprecated.

Answer 8

(a) Basal cell carcinoma
     Malignant melanoma
     Squamous cell carcinoma   3

(b) Excision for histological confirmation with adequate
     surrounding clearance. Plastic surgery may be required to

close the defect. Cryosurgery or curettage and cautery are suited for small lesions. Radiotherapy for basal cell carcinoma is an option when surgery would be poorly tolerated

Marks

4

(c) (i) Ultraviolet light on certain skin types produces dysplasia of epidermal cell layers leading to actinic keratosis; this may progress to invasive tumours

2

(ii) Wearing protective clothing and headgear; limit exposure to direct sunlight and apply sun screen lotions during exposure

1

Comment

The choice of treatment for facial lesions is based on the size of the tumour and on the physical state of the patient, as well as on cosmetic considerations. In general, surgery is preferred for those lesions that can be totally excised and the skin closed with minimal cosmetic disfigurement.

Interestingly, most melanomas occur on skin that is only intermittently exposed to the sun; individuals with higher continuous exposure have lower rates than those exposed intermittently, and curiously, the use of sunscreens may increase rather than decrease the melanoma risk. Most dysplastic lesions do not progress to skin malignancy; some may regress with time.

CHAPTER 6: ENDOCRINOLOGY, BREAST AND CHEST

Answer 1 **Marks**

(a) (i) Thyroid and parathyroid glands
Thyroglossal cyst
Cervical lymph nodes
Branchial cyst 2

(ii) Thyroid and parathyroid swellings:
move with swallowing
Thyroglossal cyst: lies over hyoid bone
Branchial cyst: lies near angle of mandible
Lymph nodes: usually lateral to mid-line 2

(b) Neck and thoracic inlet views
Ultrasound, radioisotope scan
Thyroid function tests, serum Ca^{++}
FNAB 2

(c) Thyroid cancer, or when malignancy cannot be excluded
Dyspnoea due to tracheal deviation/compression
Toxicity non-responsive to antithyroid agents
Retrosternal extension
Cosmetic considerations 4

Comment

A swelling located over the thyroid cartilage is almost invariably a goitre and requires functional assessment. Branchial and thyroglossal cysts require excision as they are liable to become infected and symptomatic. Enlarged cervical lymph nodes are caused by a host of local and systemic factors, and node biopsy may be required to assist in diagnosis or treatment. Thyroid cancers are treated surgically by total or near-total thyroidectomy, except for some anaplastic tumours and lymphomas. The latter respond well to chemotherapy, whereas in the former, the response to any form of treatment is poor.

Answer 2

(a) (i) Thyrotoxicosis 1

		Marks
(ii)	Proptosis; lid lag; lid retraction Fine tremor; rapid sleeping pulse Thyroid bruit, functional systolic murmur	3

(b) TSH, T3, T4

^{131}I thyroid scan   3

(c) Inpatient monitoring of pulse, BP and respiration
Antithyroid drugs (e.g. carbimazole)
Antiarrhythmic agents (e.g. propranolol)
Night sedation (e.g. nitrazepam)
Subtotal thyroidectomy when the patient is euthyroid
Lugol's iodine is administered for a few days pre-operatively   3

Comment

Subtotal thyroidectomy is the surgical treatment of choice for thyrotoxicosis. In the presence of eye signs the condition is referred to as Graves' disease. Eye signs rarely respond to medical measures or subtotal thyroidectomy. Orbital decompression or tarsorraphy may be required for cosmetic purposes and occasionally for conjunctivitis and chemosis.

Answer 3

(a) Texture and firmness of goitre
Retrosternal extension
Pain on palpation
Presence of palpable neck nodes suggests papillary, medullary or anaplastic tumours
Palpable bony lesions suggest follicular or anaplastic carcinoma   3

(b) Thyroid malignancy invading the larynx or the recurrent laryngeal nerve causing vocal cord palsy
Indirect laryngoscopy   2

(c) (i) Ultrasound scan of the thyroid with guided FNAB
X-ray of neck and thoracic inlet
^{131}I uptake thyroid scan   3

171

(ii) Poor or no uptake of isotope ^{131}I in a discrete area suggests absence of functional thyroid tissue. This may represent a cystic lesion or a solid lesion, e.g. a follicular adenoma or a carcinoma	**Marks** 2

Comment
Papillary carcinomas account for 60% of all thyroid malignancies and have a good prognosis, despite nodal recurrence. Lymphatic spread also occurs in medullary (C-cell) and anaplastic carcinomas but blood-borne spread is common, and the prognosis poor. Calcitonin is produced by medullary tumours and is used as a tumour marker to detect recurrence following total thyroidectomy.

Answer 4

(a) Ca^{++} and phosphate are lost from bone due to loss of renal tubular reabsorption, leading to osteoporosis   3

(b) Fall in serum Ca^{++} due to urinary loss stimulates PTH secretion and, if sustained, leads to parathyroid hyperplasia   3

(c) Removal of all parathyroid glands and place patient on long-term α-calciferol (vitamin D analogue) therapy   4

Comment
In primary hyperparathyroidism the increased PTH production is due to primary hyperplasia, an adenoma or, rarely, a carcinoma of the parathyroid. Treatment consists of removal of all four glands, when hyperplastic, with possible re-implantation of a portion of one gland in a surgically accessible site. When removing a functional adenoma or a carcinoma the other glands are usually hypoplastic and do not require removal.

Secondary hyperparathyroidism is due to a sustained low serum Ca^{++} level from any cause. Re-establishing normal serum Ca^{++} should lead to resolution of the hyperplastic state, though this is uncommon in chronic renal failure.

In tertiary hyperparathyroidism PTH production becomes independent of serum Ca^{++} levels, and the glands become autonomous, leading to hypercalcaemic states. Total parathyroidectomy and vitamin D analogue administration brings about homeostasis.

Marks

Answer 5

(a) (i) Phaeochromocytoma   1

(ii) Serum and urinary noradrenaline and/or adrenaline levels would be elevated   2

(b) (i) The catecholamines secreted by the tumour produce cardiovascular instability, i.e. hypertension and cardiac arrhythmias   2

(ii) α-blockade by phenoxybenzamine (20–80 mg daily in divided doses) lowers the BP
ß-blockade by propranolol (120–240 mg daily in divided doses) converts cardiac irregularities to sinus rhythm   3

(iii) Adrenalectomy   2

Comment

Phaeochromocytomas are neuro-ectodermal tumours of the sympathetic chain, 90% of which arise in the adrenal gland, and the remainder elsewhere along the chain. Most tumours release both adrenaline and noradrenaline but large tumours produce only noradrenaline. Scanning with ^{131}I or ^{132}I metaiodobenzylguanidine (MIBG) produces specific uptake in sites of sympathetic activity and is used for diagnostic confirmation. Adrenal surgery must be supported by α and ß blockade (the former must precede the latter) along with whole-blood transfusion as required to re-expand the contracted intravascular volume.

Answer 6

(a) (i) Cushing's disease or syndrome   1
(ii) Dexamethasone suppression test   1

	Marks
(b) (i) Pituitary gland or adrenal gland	1

(b) (ii) High resolution CT scan with IV contrast or MRI scan   1

(iii) Pituitary gland: gigantism or acromegaly
Hyperprolactinaemic syndrome
Thyrotoxicosis
Adrenal gland: phaeochromocytoma
Conn's syndrome
Addison's disease   3

(c) Medical treatment with anti-secretory drugs
Surgical removal of pituitary tumour by trans-sphenoidal
hypophysectomy
Radiotherapy if surgical excision is incomplete   3

Comment

Cushing's disease is due to an adrenocorticotropin (ACTH)-secreting pituitary tumour, resulting in bilateral adrenocortical hyperplasia and secretion of adrenal corticosteroids. Cushing's syndrome is due to an adrenal tumour or to a cortisol-secreting ectopic source, such as a bronchial carcinoma. The diagnosis of Cushing's disease is based on a failure of the pituitary source of ACTH to be suppressed by dexamethasone. Corticotrophin-releasing hormone given to those with a pituitary source of ACTH results in a normal or exaggerated corticotrophin or cortisol response, but adrenal tumours or ectopic sources of ACTH do not respond.

Answer 7

(a) (i) Express nipple discharge
Thickening/eczema of nipple; peau d'orange
Breast lump   2

(ii) Supraclavicular nodes
Axillary nodes
Liver enlargement
Contralateral breast   2

	Marks
(iii) Intraduct papilloma Ductal carcinoma *in situ* Duct ectasia	3

(b) Cytology on nipple discharge
Mammography and/or U/S scan
FNAB of a palpable lesion
Wire-guided excision biopsy   3

Comment

Duct papilloma, common between the ages of 35–50 years, usually presents with a blood-stained nipple discharge as the only symptom. On examination a lump may be felt beneath the areola. Removal of the papilloma and the involved duct (microdochectomy) or ducts (major duct excision) is curative. However, a ductal carcinoma *in situ* may have an identical clinical presentation and would necessitate a mastectomy.

Answer 8

(a) (i) Tumour size
       Skin involvement
       Pectoral fascia involvement
       Satellite lesions   2

   (ii) Axillary nodes
       Supraclavicular nodes
       Internal mammary chain
       Inferior epigastric chain   2

(b) Ultrasound
Mammogram
FNAB; excision biopsy   2

(c) Removal of the entire breast or part, with axillary nodal sampling/clearance
Radiotherapy
Chemotherapy
Hormonal manipulation   4

Comment   **Marks**

FNA cytology, ultrasonographic and mammographic findings
are graded from benign to obviously malignant. When all three
parameters show high grades for malignancy, breast ablation
may be safely undertaken. Otherwise, histological confirmation
on biopsy must be awaited. The 'frozen section biopsy, query
proceed to mastectomy' scenario is less often seen today, as a
delay of a few days between tumour biopsy and mastectomy does
not adversely alter the prognosis. Further, a 'staged mastectomy'
allows for better emotional and psychological preparation of the
patient.

Answer 9

(a) (i)   Invasive duct (scirrhous) carcinoma   1

    (ii) Palpate right axilla and supraclavicular fossa
       Examine contralateral breast and abdomen
       CXR and bone scan
       Liver scan and pelvic ultrasound examination   3

(b) (i)   Yes   1

    (ii) Wide local excision, with tamoxifen   2

    (iii) The lesion may persist unchanged for a considerable
       period of time before metastasising. It is possible she
       may die in the meantime of an unrelated cause   3

Comment

Scirrhous tumours in the elderly are usually very slow growing
and slow to metastasise. Surgical treatment, therefore, should be
confined to local removal. If surgery is declined, a course of
radiotherapy, with tamoxifen, may shrink the tumour and improve the prognosis. There is little place for adjunct chemotherapy.

Answer 10

(a) Mammography (for those >35 years of age)

	Marks
Ultrasound scan of breast (for those <35 years of age)	
FNA cytology	3

(b) LFT; CXR
   Ultrasound and/or isotope liver scan
   Radionucleide bone scan
   Bone marrow aspiration biopsy
   Brain scan (only if indicated)   3

(c) Surgical measures:
   Segmental mastectomy (if lesion is peripherally sited) or total
   mastectomy with axillary node sampling or clearance
   Radiotherapy to chest wall and/or axilla is determined by
   tumour bed biopsies and axillary nodal status
   Adjuvant chemotherapy for distant spread   4

Comment

Palpable and impalpable breast lesions may be graded by
mammography and ultrasonography as well as by cytology to
determine malignancy. If these findings are equivocal, stereotactic
guided wire localization enables impalpable lesions to be located
and removed for histology. Definitive cancer surgery should not be
performed on the basis of any one positive parameter, i.e. clinical,
cytological or imaging (positive cytology must be supported by
ultrasonography and mammography or Tru-cut biopsy). Breast-
conserving operations remove small, unifocal cancers (less than 4
cm in size). Axillary node dissection is mainly for the staging of the
disease for adjuvant therapy.

Answer 11

(a) Congenital diaphragmatic hernia   1

   Mediastinal shift to the right
   Presence of bowel and/or gastric gas shadows in left pleural
   cavity
   Collapse/compression of left lung   3

(b) Acute respiratory distress due to gastric dilatation leading to
   collapse and consolidation of the affected lung

	Marks
Volvulus of herniated stomach	
Acute bowel obstruction may lead to perforation of herniated bowel loop	3

(c) Surgical reduction of abdominal contents from the pleural cavity and excision of the herniated sac
Repair of defect in left diaphragm
Re-expansion of left lung
Ventilatory support in the postoperative period   3

Comment
The usual sites of congenital diaphragmatic herniae are the foramen of Bochdalek (pleuro-peritoneal hernia), oesophageal hiatus, foramen of Morgagni (anteriorly) and the dome. The condition must be distinguished from acute respiratory distress syndrome, oesophageal atresia and hypertrophic pyloric stenosis. Occasionally the child may present with impending or actual obstruction of the herniated bowel loop. Radiological features are, therefore, important in establishing the diagnosis.

Answer 12

(a) General anaesthesia: left lateral position with right arm supported on an arm rest
Aseptic skin preparation
Insertion of fibre-optic scope into pleural space through a stab incision
Structures visualized: lung surface, adhesions and fluid in pleural space
Pleural biopsies and fluid aspiration   3

(b) Pre-op workup, including lung function studies
Single lung anaesthesia
Thoracotomy: decortication with evacuation of inflammatory tissue and pus
Tissue samples sent for histology, and microbiological culture, including TB   4

(c) Complication of chronic lung infections, e.g. lung abscess
Organisms: TB, *Staphylococcus aureus*

	Marks
Iatrogenic introduction of infection into pleural space (during diagnostic needle aspiration)	3

Comment

The thoracoscopy would have been preceded by CXR and CT or MRI scans to localize the primary lesion in the lung. A primary tumour of the lung or pleura may give rise to these symptoms but a pyogenic or tubercular lung lesion is more common. In immunocompromised patients, chronic lung infections with atypical organisms frequently lead to pulmonary complications, such as abscess formation and empyema.

Answer 13

(a)   Papillary carcinoma of thyroid
Bronchial carcinoma
Breast carcinoma
Gastric carcinoma
Pancreatic carcinoma   2

(b)   Bronchial small cell carcinoma
CXR (postero-anterior including lateral views)
Sputum for cytology
Bronchoscopy with brush and tissue biopsies for cytology and histology, respectively
Whole body CT scan for metastases   4

(c)   Removal of primary tumour (lobectomy or pneumonectomy) and regional lymph nodes
Adjuvant chemotherapy   4

Comment

Small cell carcinomas account for 15% and squamous and adenocarcinomas for 70% of all lung cancers. Mediastinoscopy for nodal biopsies in the chest indicates the extent of nodal involvement by tumour. When contralateral nodes are involved surgery is ill-advised. Only 20% of patients with lung cancer are considered suitable for surgery. The majority receive palliation with chemotherapy.

Answer 14   **Marks**

(a) (i)   Ischaemic heart disease   1

    (ii) ECG, Echocardiogram   1

    (iii) Ischaemic changes in pre-cordial leads
       Myocardial and valvular functional defects   2

(b) Coronary angiography defines the site(s), extent and degree
of stenosis and treatment should involve balloon angioplasty
and/or insertion of coronary stents to revascularise diseased
vessels   3

(c) Coronary artery bypass grafting (CABG) of diseased vessels
using the internal mammary or the gastro-epiploic artery or
the long saphenous vein. The operation is performed by use
of extracorporeal circulation, with systemic anticoagulation   3

Comment
Balloon angioplasty and CABG have been shown to significantly
reduce myocardial infarcts in patients with critical cardiac
ischaemia. Bypass grafting is indicated when the angiogram
shows extensive narrowing of two or more coronary vessels not
amenable to angioplasty.

Answer 1

Marks

(a) (i) Pleomorphic adenoma of parotid gland

1

   (ii) Size and location
Per oral examination of fauces for involvement of deep part of gland
Involvement of branches of the facial nerve

3

(b) Contraindicated due to seeding of tumour along the needle track to skin

2

(c) (i) A conservative superficial parotidectomy (conservative total parotidectomy with preservation of the facial nerve branches if the deep part of the gland is involved)

3

   (ii) Facial nerve trunk and its five branches must be preserved

1

Comment

Pleomorphic adenomas are locally invasive and 'shelling out' of the tumour invariably leads to recurrence. Re-exploration may compromise the facial nerve and its branches. Transient facial palsy is not uncommon in the postoperative period and is due to neuropraxia from bruising or tissue swelling.

Answer 2

(a) (i) Ludwig's angina (acute cellulitis of the submandibular and cervical regions)
Inflammation and swelling of tissue planes superficial and deep to the investing layer of the deep cervical fascia, involving the submandibular region and the floor of the mouth

2

   (ii) Streptococcal species
Vincent's organisms
Gram-negative anaerobes

2

(b) (i)   The inflammatory oedema extends deep to the invest-   **Marks**
          ing layer of deep cervical fascia at and above the level   2
          of the hyoid bone, involving the glottis and displacing
          the tongue upwards and out through the mouth, leading
          to the imminent danger of asphyxiation

     (ii) Rehydration and analgesia
          IV amoxycillin or a cephalosporin with metronidazole
          gives broad spectrum therapy and usually leads to rapid
          resolution

          If resolution is delayed, surgical decompression and
          drainage of the submandibular space under local infil-
          tration anaesthesia is required   4

Comment

Ludwig's angina is an infection of a closed fascial space and, if
untreated, the inflammatory exudate may track along the stylohyoid
muscle to the submucosa of the glottis, when the patient is in
danger of asphyxiation from glottic oedema.

Surgical decompression is through a curved incision beneath the
mandible, displacing the submandibular gland and dividing the
mylohyoid muscles, thereby opening up the fascial space.

Answer 3

(a) Dysphagia for solids and/or liquids
     Pain on swallowing
     Retrosternal pain/discomfort
     Vomiting old food
     Aspirating saliva leading to recurrent chest infections
     Site of obstruction as indicated by patient   2

(b) (i)   Bulbar (and pseudobulbar) palsy
          Extra-oesophageal compression due to mediastinal
          tumours
          Iron deficiency anaemia
          Pharyngeal pouch

	Marks
Oesophageal causes:	
Scleroderma	
Inflammatory stricture	
Malignant stricture	
Achalasia	3

(ii) Barium swallow: outlines the lesion and defines the anatomical site
OGD: Visual appearance and biopsy of lesion   2

(c) Aetiology: Hiatus hernia produces reflux oesophagitis and stricture
Malignant stricture: smoking and alcohol or Barrett's oesophagus lead to squamous metaplasia and anaplasia   3

Comment

The oesophagus is inaccessible to clinical examination; consequently, a working diagnosis of oesophageal cancer must be based on the presenting symptoms and confirmed by endoscopy or imaging. Occasionally a patient may present with respiratory symptoms due to aspiration or tumour extension into the trachea or bronchus. Surgery is aimed at removing the tumour and restoring continuity by bringing the stomach up into the chest or by interposing a loop of large bowel. Radiotherapy is a viable treatment option, as squamous carcinomas are radiosensitive.

Adenocarcinomas of the gastric fundus may extend into the oesophagus, producing dysphagia. Surgery entails an oesophago-gastrectomy with reconstruction, using either the distal gastric remnant or a jejunal Roux loop.

Answer 4

(a) (i) Peptic ulcer disease   1

(ii) Stressful lifestyle
Helicobacter pylori infection
Alcohol and smoking
Irregular meals   2

(b) Oesophago-gastroduodenoscopy   **Marks**
     Sedation (0.2–5 mg IV midazolam)
     Mouth guard and anaesthetic throat spray
     Visualization through endoscope or on video screen
     Endoscopic biopsy via biopsy channel   2

(c) (i)   Adopt healthy life style measures
           Stop oral intake of anti-inflammatory agents
           Eradication of *H. pylori* by broad-spectrum antibiotics
           (amoxycillin and clarithromycin or metronidazole)
           with H_2-receptor blockade (cimetidine, ranitidine), or
           calcium channel blockade (omeprazole or lansoprazole)
           Surgery (anti-acid procedure) only on failure of medi-
           cal measures   3

     (ii) Complications of peptic ulceration: bleeding, perfora-
           tion, stenosis causing gastric outlet obstruction
           Chronic pre-pyloric ulceration may predispose to gas-
           tric carcinoma   2

Comment

The importance of stress, alcohol and tobacco in the aetiology of
this disease requires the implementation of 'life style measures'
aimed at reducing these factors and promoting health.

Since the advent of effective medical measures in ulcer healing,
surgery for peptic ulcer disease is reserved for the complications
of bleeding, perforation, stenosis and possible malignancy.

An anti-ulcer procedure involves denerving the stomach
(vagotomy) and draining the denervated stomach (by a pyloroplasty
or a gastro-enterostomy).

Answer 5

(a) (i)   Hypertrophic pyloric stenosis   2

     (ii) Achalasia of the cardia   1
           Duodenal atresia   1
           Annular pancreas

Marks

(iii) The hypertrophied pylorus ('pyloric tumour')   1

(b) Hypertrophy of the circular smooth muscle fibres of the pylorus producing a functional gastric outlet obstruction   2

(c) Medical measures: rehydration; smooth muscle relaxants (e.g. hyocine) prior to feeds
Surgery: division of all hypertrophied muscle fibres without breaching the mucosa   3

Comment
The palpation of an enlarged pylorus following a feed, with the infant preferably asleep, is diagnostic of hypertrophic stenosis and imaging is unnecessary. Medical measures are not generally successful.

Answer 6

(a) (i)   Oesophageal atresia with/without tracheo-oesophageal fistula   1

    (ii)   Gastrograffin swallow   1

(b) (i)

    (ii)   Passage of nasal feeding tube into stomach to confirm oesophageal patency by aspirating stomach contents   2

(c)   Transthoracic excision of oesophageal atresia and associ-   **Marks**
       ated tracheo-oesophageal fistula, with restoration of conti-
       nuity   2

Comment
Oesophageal atresia must be diagnosed at birth to prevent the
aspiration pneumonitis that rapidly ensues. The simple process
of passing a nasal feeding catheter and the insertion of a rectal
thermometer at birth brings to light developmental abnormalities
at each end of the alimentary tract.

Answer 7

(a)   (i)   Hiatus hernia   1

       (ii)   Herniation of portion of stomach into left pleural cavity
               leading to a sliding or rolling hernia resulting in
               oesophageal ulceration and bleeding, and later oesopha-
               geal stricture in the former. Squamous metaplasia may
               occur in the portion of stomach that slides into the
               chest, giving rise to Barrett's oesophagus, a
               premalignant condition   3

       (iii) Barium swallow or oesophogastroscopy   1

(b)   (i)   Erect and semi-recumbent posture at work and sleep
               Anti-reflux medication (alginate preparations, antac-
               ids)
               Reduce gastric acid production with H_2-receptor block-
               ade. Weight reduction   2

       (ii)   An anti-reflux operation, such as the Nissen
               fundoplication or the Leigh Collis gastroplasty per-
               formed through the abdomen, or the Belsey repair
               performed through the chest   3

Comment
Treatment of hiatus hernia is aimed at relief of symptoms. A
dramatic improvement occurs following weight reduction in
those who are overweight. Many operations have been devised as
none have been entirely satisfactory. The Nissen fundoplication

is probably the procedure most often used and may now be
performed laparoscopically.

Answer 8

(a) Test for the presence of urease (Cloe test) for evidence of
Helicobacter pylori

Haematoxylin and eosin stain for evidence of type II gastritis
and/or the presence of *H. pylori*. Suitable culture for this
organism   3

(b) (i) *Helicobacter pylori*   1

(ii) Oral therapy with amoxycillin IG twice daily and
clarithromycin 500 mg twice daily or metronidazole
400 mg three times daily for 14 days with omeprazole 20
mg or lansoprazole 30 mg daily for 28 days   3

(c) *Helicobacter pylori* is found in the presence of type II
gastritis. It raises the local pH by ammonia production and
may thereby cause mucosal damage, leading to ulceration.
The persistence of infection leads to chronicity of the ulcers
associated with it, which in gastric ulcers may predispose to
malignancy   3

Comment
Helicobacter pylori infection has been implicated in the aetiology
of peptic ulcer disease. H_2-receptor or calcium channel blockers
reduce gastric acid production, but to achieve permanent ulcer
healing, eradication of the underlying *Helicobacter pylori* infection and the chronic gastritis it produces is required.

Answer 9

(a) Immediate control of bleeding by Sangstaken–Blakemore
tube placement, or
Endoscopic sclerotherapy and IV vasopressin
If these measures fail, consider oesophageal transection or
emergency porta-systemic shunt   4

(b) Chronic liver damage (e.g. hepatitis B infection or alcohol abuse) predisposes to cirrhosis, which in turn leads to portal hypertension and variceal bleeding — **Marks** 3

(c) Three- to six-monthly follow-up oesophagoscopy and pro-phylactic sclerotherapy of recurrent varices. Long-term follow-up is mandatory — 3

Comment
Treatment of gastro-oesophageal varices is palliative unless the underlying portal hypertension is curable. Elective surgical shunts (spleno-renal, mesocaval and porta-caval) require satis-factory liver function (Child's groups A and B) to be effective. In selected cases orthopic liver transplantation has been successful.

Answer 10

(a) (i) Peritonitis due to peptic ulcer perforation — 2

    (ii) Free gas on erect abdominal X-ray, i.e. under right diaphragm and between bowel loops
Inflammatory thickening of the pro-peritoneal fat layer in the abdominal wall — 2

(b) IV analgesia and antibiotics
IV fluids; nasogastric aspiration
Consent for emergency laparotomy
Closure of perforation and peritoneal toilet
Definitive anti-ulcer surgery in selected patients — 4

(c) Stop or change anti-inflammatory agent to one less ulcergenic
Commence long-term anti-ulcer medication — 2

Comment
Emergency surgery is mandatory in a perforated viscus due to the lethal complications of peritonitis. In a young and otherwise fit patient with a peptic perforation, recurrent ulceration may be prevented by an anti-ulcer operation during the emergency surgery. Very occasionally a 'pin hole' perforation with limited peritoneal contamination may be non-surgically managed in the

expectation that the perforation would seal itself; close monitoring is then essential to assess response.

Answer 11

(a) Primary haemorrhage: during surgery, due to uncontrolled bleeding points
Reactionary haemorrhage following return to normal BP
Secondary haemorrhage occurs a few days later, due to infection

3

(b) Quarter-hourly blood pressure, pulse and respiratory rate and central venous pressure monitoring
Examination of abdominal wound and abdominal girth measurement
Resuscitation if required
Blood volume replacement
Emergency surgical re-exploration and haemostasis

4

(c) Pneumococcal infection due to fall in cell-mediated immunity
Prophylaxis: pneumovaccine
Antibiotic (penicillin V) cover for future invasive procedures

3

Comment
Post-operative bleeding from uncontrolled bleeding points into body cavities, such as the chest and abdomen, may go unnoticed until the patient lapses into oligaemic shock. Suitably placed drains assist in its early detection, and close monitoring of vital signs enables timely resuscitation and surgical control.

To preserve immunological functions of the spleen, a small portion of the spleen may be re-implanted during splenectomy for splenic trauma.

Answer 12

(a) An ulcer with slough on an indurated base and everted edges
Pain in the tongue
Salivation

	Marks
Ankyloglossia	
Dysphagia	
Inability to articulate clearly	
Alteration in the voice	
Fetor oris	
Lump in the neck due to cervical nodal spread	3

(b) Leucoplakia
Smoking
Spirits
Spices
Sepsis
Friction (from sharp edge of tooth)
Syphilis
Candidiasis   3

(c) *In situ* and small (<1 cm) tumours are excised with a 1 cm clear margin. Lesions <2 cm are treated by interstitial irradiation by use of caesium needles or iridium wire.
For lesions >2 cm external beam irradiation is used.
Large tumours with cervical nodal metastases are treated with a combination of radiotherapy and block dissection of the neck nodes.   4

Comment
Leucoplakia is regarded as a pre-cancerous condition. When causative irritants are identified and avoided, early lesions disappear. Surgical excision of cancerous lesions on the tongue is limited due to the resulting functional disability. Except for the very small lesions, all tongue cancers are treated with radiotherapy. The place of chemotherapy is undecided.

CHAPTER 8: LIVER, GALL BLADDER AND PANCREAS

Answer 1   **Marks**

(a) (i) Calculus cholecystitis   1

    (ii) Murphy's sign
        Palpable gall bladder
        Paraesthesia over the right upper quadrant and back   2

    (iii) Ultrasound scan of the gall bladder and biliary tree   1

(b) Increasing concentrations of cholesterol, bile pigments and
lecithin in the bile, with a reduction in the bile acid pool leads
to cholesterol, pigment and calcium salt super-saturation. In
the absence of glycoprotein crystallization inhibitors and
impaired gall bladder motility and/or infection, these com-
pounds crystallize to form stones   3

(c) Remove inflamed gall bladder by open or laparoscopic
cholecystectomy. During the procedure image for stones in
the biliary tree by preoperative cholangiogram and explore
the bile duct if indicated   3

Comment
The classical symptoms of cholecystitis that follow a fatty meal are
due to cholecystokinin secreted by the presence of fat in the
duodenum stimulating a diseased gall bladder to contract, usually
against a stone. Non-functioning gall bladders, despite containing
stones, may remain silent for this reason. There is, therefore, no
indication for treating asymptomatic gall stones.

Answer 2

(a) (i) Ascending cholangitis   1

    (ii) Migration of gall stones from gall bladder into bile duct
        → obstruction → biliary stasis → ascending infection   2

    (iii) Hb and WBC detect anaemia and sepsis
        LFT indicate extent of liver damage by obstruction to
        bile flow and sepsis

Serum amylase, if elevated, suggests pancreatic duct obstruction, with pancreatitis	**Marks**
Blood cultures: aerobic and anaerobic may isolate offending organism(s)	3

(b) Ultrasound and imidoacetic acid excretion scans of the liver and biliary tree

1

(c) Rehydration with IV fluids
Analgesia
Correct anaemia
Treat infection with IV antibiotics
Drain biliary tree by percutaneous transhepatic catheter, ERCP and endoscopic sphincterotomy, or surgical drainage of bile duct, with cholecystectomy

3

Comment

Cholangiohepatitis in Western societies is caused by ascending infection due to migrating gall stones obstructing the biliary tree. It is important to distinguish this from viral hepatitis, which is largely a self-limiting illness. As progressive liver damage occurs, the biliary tree must be decompressed as an emergency, by means of a transhepatic catheter. Planned surgical or endoscopic drainage should follow.

Answer 3

(a) (i) Accidental injury or ligation of the common hepatic or bile duct

1

(ii) Percutaneous transhepatic cholangiogram (PTC)

1

(iii) CXR, coagulation screen
Vitamin K prophylaxis
Blood group and cross-match

2

(b) Biliary leak causing peritonitis due to partial/complete division of the bile duct

2

		Marks
(c)	Good exposure and visualization of the surgical field	
	Identification of anatomy of Callot's triangle	
	Preoperative cholangiogram	
	T-tube drainage following accidental injury to bile duct	4

Comment

Damage to the hepatic or bile ducts during cholecystectomy is an avoidable catastrophe. Technical inexpertise, along with the occasionally encountered anomalies of the hepatic artery and ducts, account for the majority of these misadventures. During laparoscopic cholecystectomy the surgeon should, on encountering technical difficulty, convert to an open operation. Per-operative cholangiogram assists in outlining the anatomy in a difficult dissection.

Answer 4

(a)	(i)	Gall stone ileus	1

	(ii)	Chronic calculus cholecystitis leading to erosion of the gall stone into the duodenum and its passage down the small bowel, with obstruction usually in the distal ileum	1

	(iii)	Distended loops of small bowel	
		Possible radio-opaque calculus in terminal ileum	
		Air in the biliary tree	2

(b)	Nasogastric aspiration	
	Fluid and electrolyte replacement	
	Adequate analgesia	
	Emergency laparotomy and relief of obstruction with cholecystecomy	3

(c)	Ultrasound scan of gall bladder and biliary tree to confirm calculus disease and assess calibre of bile duct	
	ERCP and sphincterotomy if duct stones are present	3

Comment

Gall stone ileus is an uncommon complication of cholelithiasis and, as a history of biliary disease may not be obvious (a propor-

tion of gall stones being silent), air in the biliary tree on **Marks**
abdominal X-ray usually clarifies the diagnosis. When removing the gall bladder, it may be found to be firmly adherent to the
duodenum, and a resulting duodenal fistula may require closure.

Answer 5

(a) (i)   Acute pancreatitis

1

   (ii) Biliary calculi and alcohol abuse

1

(b) Resuscitate:
   Oxygen by face mask or nasal catheter
   IV fluids
   Pain relief
   Nasogastric aspiration
   IV broad-spectrum antibiotics

   Monitor:
   Lung function and tissue oxygenation: respiratory rate and
   arterial blood gas estimation
   Circulation: BP, pulse rate and CVP measurement
   Liver and kidney function: U&E, LFT and urine output
   Pancreatic function: blood glucose and serum and urinary
   calcium estimations

5

(c) Hypovolaemic shock
   Respiratory failure
   Renal failure
   Secondary infection
   Pseudocyst formation
   Hypocalcaemia

3

Comment
The course of acute pancreatitis is unpredictable, irrespective of
the underlying cause. In a small minority of patients the disease
is rapidly progressive, and early identification of this group
enables close monitoring and support of cardio-respiratory and
renal functions in an intensive care setting. Surgical intervention
is restricted to complications of pancreatic haemorrhage or

necrosis in fulminant disease, or of abscess or pseudo-cyst forma- **Marks**
tion in subacute disease.

Answer 6

(a) Periampullary carcinoma or bile duct carcinoma
     Pancreatic, biliary and liver imaging by ultrasound and CT
     ERCP
     Cytology on pancreatic juice and bile obtained at ERCP
     Percutaneous Tru-cut biopsy under imaging guidance   3

(b) (i) No active measures: supportive and hospice care
          Palliation by endoscopic or transhepatic stenting of
          malignant stricture
          Surgical palliation by biliary by-pass operation
          Curative surgery:
          Pancreatoduodenectomy (Whipple's operation)   3

     (ii) Poor anaesthetic or surgical risk
          Advanced primary tumour
          Local and/or regional spread of tumour   2

(c) Haemorrhage
     Wound infection
     Wound dehiscence
     Delayed wound healing
     Renal failure   2

Comment
Most ampullary and biliary tumours are beyond curative measures
on presentation and are treated palliatively. Pain is controlled by
opiates when required. Pancreatic supplements will aid digestion
and reduce weight loss. Pruritus is associated with the jaundice and
both are relieved by stenting or bypassing the obstruction.

Answer 7

(a) (i) Stress ulcer (Curling's ulcer) of the stomach or duode-
          num
          Haemobilia   1

(ii)   Stress ulcer is treated by H_2-receptor or calcium chan-   **Marks**
nel blockade

Ulcer bleeding uncontrolled by the above measures
may be treated by submucous injection of adrenaline or
laser photocoagulation

Haemobilia is due to a fistula between a hepatic vessel
and a branch of the biliary tree. It usually resolves,
otherwise angiographic embolisation of the fistula is
required   4

(b) (i)   A pancreatic fistula   1

(ii)   A fistulogram through the drainage tube or ERCP   2

(c) (i)   A leak from damage to the bile duct system   1

(ii)   An imidoacetic acid excretion scan or ERCP   1

Comment

Complications of trauma to the bile duct or pancreas usually
present late and represent unrecognized injury. Traumatic pancreatic fistulae close on supportive measures alone if continuity
of the pancreatic duct is preserved. Complete transection, however, rarely heals without surgical intervention. Pseudocyst
formation is a late complication of pancreatic injury. It resolves
either spontaneously or following ultrasound-guided aspirations, provided there is no underlying pancreatic disease.

Answer 8

(a) (i)   A clinical label when an underlying causative factor
has not been found   1

(ii)   Obsessive-compulsive neuroses
Attention-seeking behaviour patterns
Anorexia nervosa and bulimic disorders   2

(b) (i)   Chronic relapsing pancreatitis   **Marks**
           A raised serum amylase
           A normal or low serum calcium AXR may show pancre-
           atic calcification
           Abdominal U/S scan may show pancreatic calculi, fibro-
           sis or oedema   3

    (ii) Abstinence from alcohol and a low fat diet with pancre-
           atic enzyme supplementation. When pain persists, de-
           spite patient compliance, it is usually due to fibrosis of
           the duct: relief may be achieved by splanchnic nerve
           block
           Long-term pain relief using narcotic analgesics inevita-
           bly leads to habituation and drug dependency
           Surgical measures are restricted to complications such
           as chronic relapsing pancreatitis and intractable pain
           non-responsive to other measures   4

Comment

Surgery is based on pancreatographic and CT findings. If the head of the pancreas is diseased, a pancreatoduodectomy is performed, with the distal segment draining into the stomach or jejunum. Involvement of the distal segment would require a distal pancreatectomy. Occasionally the duct is grossly dilated due to stenoses, when it is opened along its length by filleting the gland, and drained into a loop of bowel (longitudinal pancreato-jejunostomy).

Answer 1 **Marks**

(a) (i) Acute bowel obstruction due to intussusception   1

    (ii) Aetiology:
Lymphoid hyperplasia in bowel wall due to weaning
and enteric viral infections; childhood leukaemias and
bowel lymphomas   2

(b) Abdominal examination:
Distention, tympanitic, increased bowel sounds
Palpable mass
PR: empty ampulla, possibly a pelvic mass; 'redcurrant jelly'
on finger stall   3

(c) (i) Barium or gastrograffin enema   1

    (ii) Under a light general anaesthetic dilute barium is
trickled into the rectum under a hydrostatic pressure
not exceeding 30 cm of water
Screening identifies the position and features of the
intussusception. The pressure is maintained for a period (not exceeding 30 minutes) before rescreening to
assess reduction of the intussusception   3

Comment

The presence of a mobile abdominal mass with 'redcurrant jelly'
stool is diagnostic of an intussusception. Diluted barium or
gastrograffin reduces the intussusception by hydrostatic pressure
and thereby avoids an operation. However, when the diagnosis is
delayed or the presentation is late, even surgical reduction may
prove difficult, due to the extensive oedema of the trapped bowel.
Further, as the intussusception progresses, the blood supply is
compromised, with infarction of the involved bowel loop.

Answer 2

(a) Infective diarrhoea
Inflammatory bowel disease
Neoplasms, i.e. benign polyps, adenocarcinoma or lymphoma   3

(b) Sigmoidoscopy (rigid or flexible), followed by barium enema   **Marks**
     or colonoscopy, with full bowel preparation
     Endoscopic mucosal biopsies   4

(c) Ascitic tap for protein content and cytology
     A low protein content would exclude an inflammatory cause,
     and the presence of neoplastic cells would suggest a dissemi-
     nated colonic cancer
     Liver ultrasound or radioisotope scan may reveal discrete
     lesions, such as a liver abscess or metastatic tumour deposits   3

Comment

Inflammatory bowel disease and bowel cancer have similar presentations. The former is incurable but compatible with a normal
life expectancy, whereas the latter has a favourable prognosis if
detected early and a dismal outcome when diagnosed late. Ulcera-
tive colitis carries a small but significant risk of cancer, which
increases with time. These patients must, therefore, be on a colon
cancer surveillance programme.

Answer 3

(a) (i)   Distended and tympanitic abdomen, minimally tender,
           with a possible palpable lesion
           Increased bowel sounds
           Empty rectum on rectal examination, with possible
           melaena on finger stall   2

     (ii) Working diagnosis: subacute colonic obstruction due to
           neoplasia or adhesions   1

(b) (i)   Plain abdominal X-ray (supine and erect)

     (ii) Features: dilated small and large bowel loops
           Presence of air/fluid levels, faecal impaction and possi-
           bly the shadow of a colonic lesion
           A barium enema should not be performed in large bowel
           obstruction   3

(c) Management: **Marks**
   FBC, U&Es, CXR, ECG
   IV rehydration
   Correct anaemia
   Nil by mouth
   Naso-gastric aspiration if necessary
   Catheterize to monitor urine output
   Group and cross-match
   IM analgesia
   Prepare for surgical relief of bowel obstruction   4

Comment

In the middle-aged and the elderly, a malignant colonic lesion must be suspected in the absence of a history of chronic constipation, inflammatory bowel disease and post-surgical adhesions. Obstructive symptoms are delayed in proximal co-lonic tumours, due to the liquid nature of their contents. These patients may, therefore, present late with anaemia and weight loss due to tumour ulceration and invasion. Early diagnosis and appropriate surgical resection, followed by radiotherapy when indicated, offers the best prognosis.

Answer 4

(a) Dilated loops of jejunum and/or ileum with air–fluid levels
   Absence of gas in bowel distal to obstruction   2

(b) (i) Assessment of dehydration and electrolyte depletion:
        tongue moisture and skin turgor
        U&E and ABG estimation for electrolyte requirement
        and acid–base balance
        Monitor naso-gastric aspirate (approx. 1000–2000/24
        hr)
        Urine normally output (approx. 1300 ml/24 hr) and
        urine osmolarity
        Insensible to fluid loss (approx. 700 ml/24 hr)   3

   (ii) Treat deficit and daily requirements by giving isotonic
        (0.9%) saline alternating with 5% dextrose or with
        one-fifth isotonic (0.18%) saline and 4.3% dextrose

		Marks

solution with additional 60–100 mmol of K⁺ per 24 hr
(the dextrose provides 400–500 calories per 24 hr)
Twice-daily haematocrit and U&Es estimation and
urine output guide the daily replacement 3

(c) Drip and suck regime
Keep patient in fluid and electrolyte balance
Failure to respond to the above measures may require
laparotomy and division of adhesions 2

Comment
The average adult requires 2000–3000 ml of water containing at
least 100 mmol of Na⁺ and 60 mmol of K⁺ daily. These requirements are increased by the degree of dehydration. However, great
care must be exercised not to over-transfuse for 'to overload the
circulation is a grievous fault, and grievously does the patient pay
for it'. If normal bowel function does not return in a few days,
parenteral alimentation (intravenous feeding) must be considered
to prevent the breakdown of body proteins.

Answer 5

(a) Hirschsprung's disease
Ano–rectal malformations (i.e. rectal atresia, rectal stenosis,
imperforate anus) 2

(b) (i) Hirschsprung's disease or primary megacolon 1

(ii) Absence of ganglion cells in nerve plexus of the large
bowel wall, leading to spasm of the involved segment
and dilatation of the normally innervated proximal loop 3

(c) (i) Barium enema shows characteristic 'funnelling' at site
of obstruction
Rectal biopsy for histological confirmation of absence
of ganglion cells and/or cholinesterase staining for
absence of acetylcholine 2

(ii) Exclusion of the aganglionic segment by a 'pull through'
operation 2

Comment   **Marks**

In Hirschsprung's disease there is a complete physiological obstruction in the distal colon at or above the peritoneal reflection. Barium enema is diagnostic and demonstrates the dilated normal proximal bowel leading to a coned transitional zone and to the narrowed segment, the aganglionic zone. Those with a very short segment of aganglionic bowel may present later in childhood or, very occasionally, in adulthood.

Answer 6

(a) (i) Exomphalos (omphalocoele)   1

    (ii) During intra-uterine life a portion of intestine lies outside the abdomen (between the 6th and 12th week) Due to an error in development, the intestine fails to return to the abdomen at birth, with a resultant defect in the abdominal wall   3

(b) Immediate surgery aimed at reducing the contents of the sac and closing the defect in the abdomen
The sac is covered with moist dressing to prevent rupture prior to surgery
If closure of the abdominal defect is not possible, a silastic sheath may be sutured on to the abdominal wall until elective repair a few weeks later   3

(c) Oesophageal atresia (with or without tracheo–oesophageal fistula)
Duodenal atesia (also intestinal atresia)
Imperforate anus (ano-rectal malformation)   3

Comment

Exomphalos is when a portion of the alimentary tract lies outside the abdominal cavity enclosed by the umbilical cord. It differs from gastroschisis, where the abdominal contents are exteriorized through a defect in the abdominal wall adjacent to the umbilical cord.

When these anomalies are associated with a large defect or a poorly developed abdominal wall, it is inadvisable to attempt to

reduce the contents and close the defect, due to ensuing respiratory **Marks**
complications. It may be possible to achieve skin cover alone, or a
silastic sheath may be sutured on to the opening and the contents
gradually reduced by twisting the sheath over a period of time as the
abdominal wall expands.

Answer 7

(a) (i)   Ischio-rectal abress   1

    (ii) Anal mucosal crypt infection which persists to form a crypt
        abscess which then enlarges and extends into peri-anal fat;
        expansion in the confined ischio-rectal fossa leads to severe
        pain   3

(b) (i)   Fistula *in ano*   1

    (ii) Incision and drainage under a general anaesthetic with
        curettage of the abscess cavity with de-roofing
        The cavity is packed with ribbon gauze soaked in antiseptic 2

    (iii) Low fistulous tracts must be excised or laid open. In high
        fistulae, i.e. those that lie above the anal sphincters, a seton
        of nylon or braided wire is threaded in and tied to gradually
        obliterate the tract. Complicated or recurrent high fistulae
        may require excision, with preliminary faecal diversion   3

Comment
Ischio-rectal abscess must be surgically drained on presentation. The
presence of Gram-negative coliform organisms in the pus obtained
suggests communication with the bowel. However, effective surgical
measures prevent the formation of sinuses or fistulae. Complicated
fistulae are the result of recurrent peri-anal abscess formation and
form tortuous tracts with multiple cutaneous openings. These require
staged surgical procedures for a cure, with a preliminary colostomy.

Answer 8

(a) (i)   Digital rectal examination to palpate lesions in the rectum
        and pelvis

			Marks
		Rigid sigmoidoscopy to visualise the rectum and distal sigmoid colon	
		Protoscopy to visualise the ano-rectum	3
	(ii)	Carcinoma	
		Ulcerative colitis	
		Crohn's colitis	
		Polyps	3
(b)	(i)	Prolapsing haemorrhoids	
		(Other causes are ano-rectal polyps and mucosal pro-lapse)	1
	(ii)	Injection sclerotherapy	
		Rubber banding	
		Haemorrhoidectomy	
		Cryosurgery	
		(and stretch)	3

Comment

Rectal bleeding in any form should alert the clinician to the possibility of a large bowel tumour, especially in the older age group. The presence of piles (the commonest cause of bleeding PR) should not preclude a sigmoidoscopic examination, as the piles may prove to be a red herring masking a more sinister proximal lesion. In the presence of a recent alteration in bowel habit with or without weight loss, imaging of the entire colon or colonoscopy may be required to exclude an occult neoplasm.

Answer 9

(a)	(i)	General appearance: size, shape, contact bleeding, punched out, shallow or irregular	
		Base: indurated or soft, fixed or mobile	
		Edges: everted, rolled up or sloping	3
	(ii)	Multiple punch biopsies from the ulcer edge	2
(b)	(i)	Liver	1

(ii) Ultrasound or radio-isotope scan of the liver   1

(iii) Pre-operative bowel preparation
      An anterior resection of the rectum and distal sigmoid
      colon preserving the anal canal if the tumour is above the
      peritoneal reflection, or a synchronised combined abdomino-
      perineal excision of the ano-rectum and distal sigmoid
      colon if the anal canal is involved   3

Comment
It is necessary to counsel the patient regarding the planned operation
and the need for either a temporary or permanent colostomy, its siting
and management. Sphincter-preserving operations for rectal cancer
aim at restoring bowel continuity, thereby avoiding a permanent
stoma of an abdomino-perineal excision. However, a 5 cm distal
clearance of the tumour must be attainable to avoid tumour recurrence
at the anastomosis.

Answer 1   **Marks**

(a) (i) Testis, epididymis, cord structures
        Tunica vaginalis, scrotal skin
        Abdominal hernial contents   3

    (ii) Examination:
         Get above it to exclude hernia
         Feel for the epididymis, cord and testis and examine for
         a hydrocele   2

(b) (i) Teratoma, seminoma, yolk sac tumour   3

    (ii) Orchidectomy
         Radiotherapy to para-aortic nodes
         Chemotherapy   2

Comment

Scrotal swellings include vaginal hydrocele (most common), tuberculosis and tumour. Epididymo-orchitis, due to pyogenic organisms, generally have an acute presentation. When a testicular tumour is suspected, percutaneous biopsy is contraindicated due to seeding of tumour in the needle track, with spread to the groin nodes. An open biopsy with frozen section histology and proceed to orchidectomy if malignancy is confirmed.

Answer 2

(a) Right reducible inguinal or femoral hernia
    Visible or tactile cough impulse above or below the inguinal
    ligament   3

(b) Prostatic enlargement or urethral stricture
    Palpable urinary bladder
    Enlarged prostate on PR, or palpable stricture in penile
    urethra   3

(c) Investigate urinary symptoms with flow studies IVU and/or
    ultrasound of urinary tract; urethro-cystoscopy

Treatment:	**Marks**
Prostatectomy or stricturoplasty and hernia repair	4

Comment

Chronic increase in intra-abdominal pressure may precipitate an abdominal hernia. Chronic obstructive airway disease, chronic constipation, ascites or an obstructive uropathy must be excluded in patients presenting with a groin hernia and the precipitating cause(s) treated before the hernia is repaired. Otherwise recurrence is almost inevitable.

Answer 3

(a) (i) Torsion of the spermatic cord (testis)   1

    (ii) Pyrexia; tender, swollen testis, horizontal lie of testis 'dumbell sign'
Absent urethral discharge
Clear urine   3

(b) Surgical exploration with orchiopexy, if testis is non-viable perform an orchidectomy
Fix the other testis to prevent it torting   3

(c) Exploration is no longer indicated due to testicular non-viability
Antibiotics and analgesics
Observe in the ward until symptoms resolve
Testicular atrophy is the end result
The opposite testis must be fixed at an early date   3

Comment

An attempt may be made to untwist a torted testis on presentation; the immediate relief of pain indicates success. Surgical fixation should then be performed without undue delay. The opposite testis is also fixed, as the anatomical abnormality is likely to be bilateral.

Answer 4 **Marks**

(a) (i) Pneumaturia 1

    (ii) Colo-vesical or colo-uteric fistula caused by either invasion of the urinary bladder or ureter by recurrent tumour or radiation damage 2

(b) Intravenous urography
Cytoscopy
Cystourethrogram 3

(c) Diverticular disease
Crohn's disease
Bladder cancer
Diabetes mellitus 4

Comment

Closure of the fistula is usually not possible when it is due to tumour infiltration or in the presence of post-irradiation fibrosis. Faecal diversion by fashioning a proximal defunctioning colostomy halts further contamination of the renal tract with bowel pathogens. It also facililates further irradiation of the pelvis for tumour recurrence without the risk of radiation colitis.

Answer 5

(a) Early:
Haemorrhage
Clot retention
Infection
Water intoxication

    Late:
Urethral stricture
Recurrent obstruction due to prostate regrowth
Incontinence 4

(b) Myoadenomatous hyperplasia
Prostatic carcinoma 2

		Marks
(c)	Bladder outflow obstruction leads to chronic retention of urine, which produces hydronephrosis and atrophy of the renal cortext, due to pressure effects and infection	
	Prostatic cancer, when present (incidence 25% at 75 years of age), invades the capsule and may involve the pelvis with bony metastases or the rectum with fistula formation	4

Comment

Haemorrhage following prostatic surgery is usually reactionary, leading to clot retention; or secondary (usually a week after the operation) due to infection or straining. Perforation of the bladder or breaching the prostatic capsule may occur during transurethral surgery and, if not immediately recognized, leads to severe haemorrhage from the prostatic venous plexus in the latter. Bladder perforation may be undetected postoperatively due to the indwelling catheter preventing extravasation of urine. Both these complications are serious and may require re-exploration under a general anaesthetic.

Answer 6

(a)	Diabetic neuropathy Psychosexual dysfunction Undescended testes Previous pelvic surgery or injury	3
(b)	Sperm count Sperm motility Percentage of normal to abnormal cells pH and sugar content of seminal fluid	3
(c)	Tuberculous epididymo-orchitis	1
	Urinalysis: microscopy and culture for tubercular bacilli Testicular biopsy for histological and microbiological evidence of tuberculosis	3

Comment

An obvious cause of sterility is previous vasectomy and a request for surgical reversal is made on presentation. Surgical proce-

dures for erectile dysfunction vary from penile revascularization **Marks**
to the insertion of prostheses.

Answer 7

(a) Acute tubular necrosis
Acute rejection
Obstruction of the collecting system
Infarction of transplant   2

(b) Daily serum U&E
Isotope renography for state of perfusion
Ultrasonography – reveals urinary tract obstruction,
haematoma, urinoma, and renal artery flow
Percutaneous renal biopsy to diagnose acute tubular necrosis
or acute rejection   3

(c) (i) Cyclosporin A and/or azathioprine, anti-thymocyte
globulin and prednisolone   2

(ii) Increased incidence of malignancies, i.e. with
azathioprine immunosuppression, e.g. tumours of
reticuloendothelial system, central nervous system
and skin

Increased incidence of upper GI bleeding with high
doses of steroids   3

Comment

Oliguria or anuria due to acute tubular necrosis occurs immediately post-transplantation, the extent of the tubular damage is
dependent on the warm ischaemia time of the donor kidney.
Dialysis must be continued until the kidney recovers. Rejection of
the donor organ may be acute (within three months) or chronic
(thereafter), with progressive impairment of urine production.
The former responds favourably to anti-rejection therapy.

Answer 8

(a) (i) Pelvi-ureteric colic due to renal calculus disease   1

	Marks
(ii) Test urine for red blood cells	2

(b) Adequate analgesia
Plain abdominal X-ray and IVU to establish site of
calculus
If calculus is <5 mm in size await spontaneous passage
If calculus is >5 mm in size cystoscopic basket extraction,
if in lower third of ureter, or cysto-ureterotomy if impacted
in intravesical portion of distal ureter
Shock-wave lithotripsy or operative removal may be indicated for stones in the renal pelvis and proximal ureter   5

(c) Hereditary and acquired defects in calcium and phosphate
metabolism
Hyperparathyroidism
Hyperoxaluria
Cystinuria   2

Comment
The need for open surgery for renal stones has been largely
replaced by endoscopic or percutaneous extraction and by extracorporeal shock-wave lithotripsy. Ureteric cathetcrization and
irrigation frequently enable impacted uteric calculi to pass;
occasionally those impacted above the pelvic brim may be
pushed up into the renal pelvis and fragmented or extracted
percutaneously. Leaking abdominal aneurysms may mimic renal colic and are rapidly fatal unless promptly resuscitated and
operated upon.

Answer 9

(a) (i) Hydronephrosis
Cystic kidney
Nephroblastoma (Wilms' tumour)
Mesoblastic nephroma   2

(ii) Ultrasound
CT and/or MRI scans of the abdomen

	Marks
IVU	
Renal angiography	3

(b) (i) CXR
        Liver scan
        Bone scan
        Bone marrow biopsy   2

    (ii) Surgical: Radical nephroureterectomy

        Radiotherapy: Pre- and/or post-operative courses

        Chemotherapy: Childhood tumours of the kidney or adjacent neuroectoderm are chemosensitive and respond well to a combination of two or more agents   3

Comment

Nephroblastomas and neuroblastomas usually present with a palpable loin swelling and anaemia. Both lesions, as well as the rarer mesoblastoma of the kidney, require radical excision.

Radiotherapy may be given prior to surgery to reduce the tumour bulk, and a post-operative course is usual. Chemotherapeutic drugs used are usually a combination of actinomycin D and vincristine or cyclophosphamide and doxorubicin or cisplatin.

Answer 10

(a) Urethral stricture

    Inflammatory – chronic urethritis (e.g. venereal infection)
    Traumatic – perineal injury producing partial rupture or ischaemic damage
    Iatrogenic – following urethral instrumentation or prostatic surgery in the older male   3

(b) Urinary retention leads to bladder diverticulae, hydroureter and hydronephrosis
    Proximal urethral diverticulum leads to periurethral abscess and urethral fisulae (watering can perineum)

	Marks
Increased abdominal pressure of straining gives rise to groin herniae, piles and rectal prolapse	3

(c) Intermittent urethral dilatation with gum-elastic bougies, either separate or filiform with screw-on followers
Self-dilatation with soft Nelaton catheters

Urethrotomy under direct vision using an optical urethrotome

Urethroplasty by excision of stricture and end-to-end anastomosis or grafting following excision of more extensive strictures   4

Comment
Gonococcal urethritis must be actively treated with antibiotics, with the prevention of re-exposure. Ineffective treatment may lead to spread of infection to produce posterior urethritis, prostatitis, epididymo-orchitis or periurethral abscess. Dilatation of urethral strictures may introduce infection manifesting as septicaemia; aseptic technique is, therefore, essential.

Answer 11

(a) Stress incontinence is caused by sphincter weakness and produces urinary leakage as a result of increased intra-abdominal pressure

Causes: Weakness of distal sphincter mechanism combined with laxity of pelvic floor musculature due to complicated or neglected labour or multiple pregnancies
Neurogenic bladder dysfunction due to demyelinating diseases (myelodysplasia, multiple sclerosis, syringomyelia)   3

(b) Exercise testing with 300 ml of fluid in bladder and measure resulting fluid loss (in the order of 10–50 ml)

Pressure–flow studies record bladder pressure and flow rate during micturition (distinguishes between genuine stress incontinence and detrusor instability)   3

(c)   Minor degrees of stress incontinence can be controlled by   **Marks**
      improving the tone of the pelvic floor musculature by pelvic
      floor exercises
      Surgical measures: colposuspension (suspending the vagi-
      nal fascia on either side of the bladder neck to the ileopubic
      ligaments)
      Neurogenic bladder dysfunction may require implantation of
      an artificial, battery-operated urinary sphincter   4

Comment

It is important to distinguish stress incontinence from idiopathic
detrusor muscle instability, as the outcome of surgery is significantly worse in the latter. The mainstay of treatment in the latter
is the use of anticholinergic agents. Symptoms of stress incontinence due to neurogenic bladder dysfunction may progress to
complete incontinence or to retention as the disease progresses.

CHAPTER 11: VASCULAR SURGERY

Answer 1

(a) Diagnosis: acute limb ischaemi due to left common femoral
arterial occlusion

Aetiological factors:
Atrial fibrillation leading to embolism
Thrombus on a previously diseased artery
Aortic dissection

3

(b) Pallor and/or skin mottling
Cold, pulselessness and pain
Reduced skin sensation
Loss of function (toes cannot be moved)
Venous guttering

3

(c) Emergency surgical work-up:
FBC, U&E, CXR, ECG, urethral catheterization
Group and cross-match 4 units

Treat as acute or acute-on-chronic occlusion with systemic
anticoagulation, aterial embolectomy or thrombectomy,
with peroperative angiogram
In some instances thromboembolytic therapy may avoid
surgery

4

Comment

Acute limb ischaemia is a surgical emergency. Systemic
heparinization (35,000–45,000 units per 24 hr) is commenced,
and thrombo-embolectomy performed with Fogarty balloon
catheters. Occasionally, thrombolysis may be achieved with
fibrinolytic agents, such as streptokinase or tissue plasminogen
activator (TPA), which is infused intra-arterially. Long-term
warfarin therapy must be commenced or the precipitating cause
treated to prevent recurrence.

Answer 2

(a) (i) Peripheral vascular disease producing stenosis of
the arteries of the right lower limb

		Marks
	Right common femoral artery or superficial and profunda femoral arteries	2

(ii) Pathogenesis of atherosclerosis: adherent microthrombi and subintimal fatty deposition lead to atheromatous plaque with or without calcification; plaque haemorrhage leads to intimal ulceration; thrombi form on the ulcerated surface, giving rise to microemboli   3

(b) Smoking
Diabetes mellitus
Hypercholesterolaemia/high fat intake
Hypertension
Family history   2

(c) Stop smoking
Close monitoring of diabetes/hypertension
Exercise to develop collateral circulation, weight reduction, low cholesterol diet
Foot care: chiropody, protective footwear, heel raise   3

Comment

Claudication can usually be distinguished from musculo-skeletal symptoms in the lower limb from the history of exercise-related pain. Peripheral vascular disease is generalized in nature, and the carotid arteries and the aorta must be clinically assessed for occult lesions. The nutritional state of the affected foot, namely skin changes and brachial–ankle pressure indices, form part of the initial assessment.

Answer 3

(a) Pale, cold limb with loss of sensation, ischaemic skin changes
Reduced or absent femoral, popliteal, dorsalis pedis, posterior tibial
Reduced ankle–brachial pressure indices
Neurological problems:
Sensation, tone, power and reflexes with muscle wasting   4

(b) (i) Retrograde transfemoral aortography   1

			Marks
	(ii)	Angioplasty of stenotic arterial lesions Focal intra-arterial infusion of prostaglandin derivative for pain relief	2

(c)   Removal of arterial occlusive disease by endarterectomy
Bypass of occlusion using native vein or synthetic vascular
grafts   3

Comment
The presence of rest pain and brachial–ankle pressure index of
>0.5 suggest critical ischaemia. Pain usually involve the leg and
foot, and there may be sensory or motor signs. Vascular reconstruction is usually required for limb salvage. However, in the
presence of distal vessel disease, unresponsive to angioplasty or
surgery, lumbar sympathectomy may improve skin perfusion.

Answer 4

(a)   Claudication or rest pain extending up to the buttock
Weak or absent distal pulses
Low resting and exercise brachial–ankle pressure indices
Loss of muscle power   3

(b)   (i)   Thrombosis, dislodgement of atheromatous plaque, or
intimal dissection during or following angioplasty
producing arterial occlusion   2

     (ii) Analgesia; anticoagulation with IV heparin
Infusion of prostaglandin-derived thrombolytic agent
Thrombo-embolectomy; removal of intimal flap   3

(c)   Smoking
Diabetes mellitus
Hyperlipidaemia/high fat intake
Hypertension
Family history   2

Comment
Vascular imaging and interventional procedures are common in
cardiology and vascular units. Complications arising therefrom,

though uncommon, may require urgent surgical intervention. Patients who are admitted for these procedures must, therefore, be adequately assessed and prepared with informed consent for such eventualities.

Marks

Answer 5

(a) (i)   False aneurysm of femoral artery   1

    (ii) Duplex Doppler scan   1

    (iii) By pressure occlusion or, failing this, by surgical repair
         of arterial wall defect   2

(b) (i)   Thrombosis, embolus, intimal plaque formation, intimal
         dissection   2

    (ii) Embolectomy/thrombectomy under imaging; intimal
         repair   4

Comment
Fibrinolytic therapy may lead to recanalization following angiographic assessment of the site of thrombotic occlusion.

A false aneurysm is a pulsatile haematoma produced by bleeding from the arterial puncture. Rarely, the adjacent femoral vein may be injured, with the formation of a traumatic arteriovenous fistula. This also presents as a pulsatile groin swelling. If detected early the fistula may be closed off by pressure occlusion with a Doppler probe. If allowed to mature it may require surgical repair.

Answer 6

(a) (i)   Abdominal aortic aneurysm   1

    (ii) Atherosclerotic changes to vessel wall with intimal
         ulceration and destruction of elastic and muscle coats
         with intraluminal thrombus formation   2

(b) Abdominal ultrasound scan   1

(c) (i)   Aneurysms <6 cm in diameter and asymptomatic –   **Marks**
      keep under surveillance
      Aneurysms >6 cm in diameter – inlay of synthetic graft   3

   (ii) Pre-operative work-up:
      CXR, FBC
      ECG
      Renal function assessment
      Hypertension control

      Group and cross-match 6–8 units of blood   3

Comment

Abdominal aneurysms over 6 cm in diameter expand progressively over time, increasing the incidence of rupture or leakage. Elective surgery is aimed at obviating this risk, as survival following rupture is small. The risks from rupture of aneurysms <6 cm equate to those of surgery: therefore a conservative approach is followed, provided the patient is kept under surveillance.

Answer 7

(a) (i)   Rupture of abdominal aortic aneurysm   1

   (ii) Resuscitation:
      Maintain airway, administer O_2
      Central and peripheral venous access
      FBC and ABG
      IV analgesia
      Group and emergency cross-match for 10–15 units of
      blood
      Monitor pulse, BP and respiration quarter-hourly
      Volume replacement with crystalloids and plasma
      expanders, and with blood when available
      Catheterize and monitor urine output
      Inform the surgical and anaesthetic teams and the
      theatre in preparation for emergency surgery
      CXR, AXR and ECG (if time permits)
      Consent patient for emergency abdominal surgery   3

	Marks
(b) Emergency Dacron graft inlay of ruptured aortic aneurysm	1

(c) (i) Spontaneous retroperitoneal haemorrhage due to over-anticoagulation 2

(ii) IV analgesia
Stop warfarin therapy
Resuscitation and replace blood volume
Administer coagulation factors in the form of fresh frozen plasma and platelet concentrates 3

Comment

It is vital to distinguish on presentation from a ruptured or leaking aneurysm left-sided pelvi-ureteric colic or diverticulitis of the left colon. Occasionally, retrosternal radiation of pain, coupled with circulatory collapse may simulate myocardial infarction. A pulsatile and expansile abdominal mass and weak or absent femoral pulses must be sought on examining the abdomen. Surgical survival is determined largely by the duration of hypotension (the interval between rupture and surgical control), this determines the incidence of cardio-respiratory complications and coagulation disorders in the peri- and post-operative periods.

Answer 8

(a) (i) Stenosis of the right internal carotid artery 1

(ii) Hypertension, diabetes mellitus, smoking, hyperlipidaemia, family history 2

(b) (i) Bilateral carotid angiography 1

(ii) Site and extent of atheromatous disease of the carotid and intracranial arteries, and cross-perfusion between the two hemispheres 2

(c) Treat pre-existing cardiac disease and/or hypertension; control diabetes mellitus
Treat hyperlipidaemia

			Marks
Right carotid endarterectomy			
Post-operatively systolic pressure to be kept below 100 mmHg			4

Comment

Atherosclerotic narrowing or ulceration is generally widespread despite symptoms being confined to one anatomic region, supplied by one or more diseased vessels. There is, therefore, the need to assess the contralateral carotid supply, myocardial and renal function, and the presence of other risk factors for stroke before planning surgery.

Answer 9

(a) Venous and vasculitic ulcers are caused by skin breakdown, due to poor nutrition
Venous bleeding follows the erosion of the ulcer into an adjacent or underlying varicosity   **3**

(b) Tourniquets are to be avoided in first aid as they cause venous congestion and increased blood loss by only occluding venous return
Venous haemorrhage is readily controlled by elevation of the affected limb and a pressure dressing   **3**

(c) Control local oedema by graduated support stockings and limb elevation when at rest
Appropriate topical ulcer treatment until healing
Surgical removal of the underlying varices   **4**

Comment

Tourniquets can cause exsanguination by preventing venous outflow but not arterial inflow. Tourniquets tight enough to occlude the latter may cause vascular damage and thrombosis. Nerve conduction injury may also occur and, if applied for a number of hours, may produce muscle necrosis and precipitate renal failure. Arterial tourniquet is used for some surgical procedures, but should not be left in place for more than an hour.

Answer 10   **Marks**

(a) (i) Venous ulcer caused by underlying venous incompe-   1
          tence

    (ii) Indolent, shallow and moist granulating floor with
         associated varicosities and surrounding pigmentation
         Induration and pitting oedema leads to poor skin nutri-
         tion   2

(b) (i) Limb elevation; daily wound toilet and non-stick dress-
         ing
         Split-skin grafting if required   2

    (ii) Treat the associated varicose veins surgically following
         ulcer healing   1

(c) Ischaemic ulcers: caused by poor tissue perfusion due to
     pressure (decubitus ulcers), atherosclerotic or diabetic vascu-
     lar occlusive disease
     Neuropathic ulcers are anaesthetic and are caused by periph-
     eral nerve degeneration, as in leprosy and diabetic neuritis
     Tropical ulcers are due to chronic skin infections caused by
     bacteria (*Mycobacterium ulcerans* causes Buruli ulcer) or
     fungi (actinomycosis, mycetoma)   4

Comment
Ulcers due to vascular diseases are painful; the exceptions being
pressure ulcers and diabetic ulcers where nerve damage occurs
alongside the ischaemic changes.

Venous ulcers in the leg may extend and become circumferential,
thereby endangering the viability of the limb. Chronicity may give
rise to squamous cell carcinoma (Marjolin's ulcer); biopsy should
be undertaken when in doubt.

Answer 11

(a) Increase in body temperature and pulse
     Increase in limb diameter and warmth

Tenderness on palpation, with or without induration	**Marks**
Postive Homans' sign	3

(b) (i) Deep vein thrombosis (DVT) of calf and/or thigh   1

    (ii) Venous stasis leads to the following sequence: DVT, pulmonary embolus, fall in pulmonary arterial supply, with consequent fall in gaseous exchange, fall in cardiac output and cardiac arrest   3

(c) Management of DVT:
Colour flow duplex imaging confirms DVT and its proximal extent. (Venogram gives further information on the iliac veins.)
IV heparin infusion of 30,000–40,000 IU/24 hr
Commence long-term warfarin therapy before discharge; monitor anticoagulation profile periodically   3

Comment
In young patients, in addition to known risk factors, such as oral contraception and smoking, spontaneous venous thrombosis may be associated with deficiencies in the coagulation profile, i.e. protein C, protein S and antithrombin III. Thrombosis of the common femoral vein with an associated lymphangitis produces a very swollen 'white leg' (phlegmasia alba dolens); extensive thrombosis of the iliac and pelvic veins produces venous obstruction and a 'blue leg' (phlegmasia caerulea dolens). In the latter, venous gangrene may threaten limb viability.

Answer 12

(a) (i) Pulmonary embolus   1

    (ii) ECG
Ventilation/perfusion scan
ABG   2

(b) Resuscitation
Analgesia
Anticoagulation

Swan–Ganz catheter to measure pulmonary artery wedge **Marks**
pressure and for selective thrombolysis
Surgical embolectomy if cardiorespiratory function dete-
riorates   5

(c) Stop smoking; avoid oral contraception
     Compression stockings
     Early mobilization
     Heparin prophylaxis   2

Comment

Pulmonary emboli originate from thrombus in the veins of the
pelvis or lower limbs. The latter may give rise to local symptoms
and/or signs and signal an impending catastrophe. Deep venous
thrombosis must, therefore, be actively treated with immediate
systemic anticoagulation. Thrombosis in pelvic veins extending
to the inferior vena cava may require angiographic placement of
a filter above it to prevent embolization.

SECTION III:
ESSAY WRITING

QUESTION 1

Write an essay on the diagnosis and treatment of primary skin cancers.

Plan

Types of skin cancer:
    Rodent cancer
    Melanoma
    Squamous cell carcinoma
    Kaposi's sarcoma

Initiating factors (if any)

Diagnosis:
    History – duration, scabbing/bleeding, pain, etc.
    Site and size
    Appearance – surface, edges, base
    Histology
    Regional lymphadenopathy

Treatment:
    Surgical – wide local excision (except Kaposi's)
    Block dissection of involved regional nodes
    Adjuvant – radio-, chemo-, immunotherapies

Prognosis:
    Dependent on type, histological grading and spread (nodal/visceral)

Follow-up:
    Long term for all except rodent ulcers
    Treatment of recurrences

QUESTION 2

Write an essay on the management of a 36-year-old man who sustained a spinal injury at C7–T1 level in a riding accident.

Plan

Immediate measures:
>Airway maintenance
>BP, pulse and respiratory monitoring
>Resuscitation, if required
>Support spine for transport

Assessment of injuries:
>Neurological examination
>Associated injuries

Treatment:
>Surgical – stabilize spinal fracture/dislocation
>Supportive – maintenance of bodily function:
>>nutrition
>>bladder
>>bowel
>
>Monitor recovery of neurological function
>Avoid morbidity: viz, bed sores, bone demineralization, muscle atrophy
>Physiotherapy – maximize functional recovery by exercise regimes and physical aids
>Community care – adjustments to home/work environment
>Long-term complications of paraplegia

QUESTION 3

A 30-year-old woman presents with an asymptomatic lump in her left breast. Discuss your clinical assessment and management.

Plan

Working diagnosis on history and clinical features

Investigations:
    Mammogram/ultrasound scan
    FNAB
    Biopsy (excisional/incisional)
    Further investigations, e.g. CXR, bone and liver scans, if indicated

Definitive diagnosis from above

Counselling of patient

Treatment:
    Surgical:
        benign – local excision
        malignant – mastectomy (segmental or total)
        axillary dissection
    Adjuvant therapy:
        based on histological type and spread:
        regional DXT
        tamoxifen
        chemotherapy
        endocrine ablation (oophorectomy, adrenalectomy, hypophysectomy)

Follow up:
    Long term (annual after five years' recurrence-free)
    Diagnosis, re-staging and treatment of recurrent disease

QUESTION 4

Write an essay on the causes, presentation and treatment of obstructive jaundice.

Plan

Causes:
    Congenital – biliary atresia
    Inflammatory – sclerosing cholangitis
    Infective – ascending cholangitis; parasitic (round) worms
    Metabolic – duct stones or sludge
    Iatrogenic – bile duct injury
    Neoplastic – cholangiocarcinoma; periampulatory carcinoma, metatastic spread to lymph nodes in portahepatitis

Presentation:
    Symptoms – weakness, loss of appetite, fever, itchiness, pale stools
    Signs – jaundice, hepatomegaly, ascites, palpable gall bladder

Treatment:
    Relief of obstruction:
    By percutaneous trans-hepatic drainage and cholangiogram and/or ERCP to identify lesion
    Antibiotic therapy on bile culture
    Surgical measures:
    Duct exploration, resection, biliary bypass
    Endoscopic stenting with/without chemotherapy for inoperable lesions

QUESTION 5

Write an essay on the causation and the diagnosis of blood in the urine in a 70-year-old man.

Plan

Causes:
    Kidneys – acute nephritis, stone, tumour
    Ureter – stone, tumour
    Bladder – acute cystitis, polyps, tumour, stone (schistosomiasis)
    Prostate – tumour, prostatic surgery
    Urethra – stone
    Unknown aetiology

History:
    Duration of haematuria
    Blood mixed in urine or appears at start/end of micturition
    Stranguary
    Abdominal symptoms, if any

Clinical findings:
    General – pallor, BP, pulse
    Renal/bladder mass
    Prostatic enlargement
    Urethral lesion

Investigations:
    FBC, U&Es
    MSU to confirm haematuria and to test for sugar
    Ultrasound scan of kidneys/bladder
    IVU
    If the above are negative/normal – repeat urinary microscopy
    If haematuria persists – uteric catherization for selective urine samples
    Renal imaging
    Once lesion is identified – histological confirmation by endoscopic biopsy
    or FNAB under imaging

QUESTION 6

Write an essay on the causation, presentation and treatment of small bowel obstruction.

Plan

Causes:
> Intraluminal – bolus obstruction
> In bowel wall – lymphoid hyperplasia and tumours leading to intussusception, vascular occulsion (mesenteric infarction)
> Extraneous – internal herniations; external hernias
> Iatrogenic – surgical adhesions or incisional herniae

Presentation:
> Symptoms and signs of complete/incomplete obstruction, viz vomiting, dehydration, constipation, colic, abdominal signs
> Characteristics of palpable mass or visible peristalsis
> Signs of bowel ischaemia

Abdominal X-ray:
> Air–fluid levels, level of obstruction from the configuration of proximal distended loops

Treatment:
> Nasogastric suction
> Rehydrate, electrolyte replacement
> Urgent surgical relief of obstruction, except in adhesion obstruction when non-surgical measures are continued
> Repair of causative hernia at same time

CHAPTER 2: MODEL ESSAYS

QUESTION:

Write an essay on the presentation and management of chronic arterial disease of the lower limb.

ANSWER 1 – A COMFORTABLE PASS

Introduction
Chronic arterial disease afflicting the aorta, the iliacs and vessels in the lower limb may produce stenosis, occlusion or aneurysmal dilatation. Atherosclerosis is the common vascular lesion and may also involve coronary, cerebral and renal arteries. Association risk factors are diabetes mellitus, hypertension, smoking, raised blood lipid levels and a family history of vascular disease.

Symptoms and signs
Stenosis of the main arteries reduces the blood flow to the lower limb producing intermittent claudication due to temporary muscle ischaemia: the claudication distance is the distance the patient is able to walk before stopping. Rest pain in the limb indicates severe restriction to blood flow, which is inadequate for resting tissue metabolism. The pain is characteristically in the foot, worse at night and relieved by dangling the limb out of bed or sleeping in a chair. Pain referred to the limb from degenerative disease of the lumbo-sacral spine, the hip or the knee or due to peripheral neuropathy must be distinguished from ischaemic pain.

Coldness, numbness and paraesthesia are present with skin pallor on elevating and duskiness on lowering the limb. Buerger's angle is the angle of elevation at which blanching first occurs and is accompanied by venous emptying or, in severe ischaemia, venous guttering. The time taken for the veins to refill on hanging the limb down indicates the extent of vascular compromise. In severe ischaemia the skin may be mottled and without sensation. Occasionally, symptoms and signs of acute-on-chronic ischaemia develop.

Ulceration occurs with severe arterial insufficiency and presents as painful, indolent, non-healing ulcers in the toes or pressure areas in the foot and occasionally over the ankle or the shin. Arterial pulses are reduced or absent distal to the diseased artery and occasionally a thrill or a bruit may be detected over the latter, caused by turbulent flow.

The presence of a pulsatile and expansile swelling in the abdomen indicates an aortic aneurysm, whereas a femoral or a popliteal aneurysm may be felt in the groin or behind the knee. They may be asymptomatic but can present with acute rupture or thrombosis.

Investigations
The severity of the symptoms determines the need for vascular investigations, and non-invasive ultrasound tests are performed routinely on presentation. The ankle–brachial pressure index is the ratio of systolic pressure in the ankle to that in the arm. The normal is 1.0. In claudicants the resting index is usually <1.0 and falls below the resting value following exercise. A resting index of ≤0.5 indicates critical ischaemia. The results of non-invasive tests indicate the need for further assessment with a view to treatment. Angiography by conventional or digital techniques demonstrates the anatomical site or sites and the severity of the disease process and enables treatment to be planned.

Treatment
Most claudicants require only reassurance and advice regarding weight reduction, low fat diet and stopping smoking, as appropriate. Intercurrent diseases, such as diabetes and hypertension, must be actively treated. Daily exercise regimes to improve the blood supply by developing collateral circulations must be actively encouraged. Foot care is essential to avoid injury to skin that may already be compromised. A daily aspirin tablet (75 mg) improves tissue perfusion by lowering the blood viscoscity.

In the presence of incapacitating claudication or rest pain, transluminal angioplasty is used as the first line of treatment. It dilates the stenosed lumen with an inflatable balloon introduced on an arterial catheter under fluoroscopic screening. Intraluminal stents may occasionally be inserted to keep the lumen open following dilatation.

Surgery for occlusive disease is indicated when angioplasty is not feasible. Aortic or aorto–iliac disease may be bypassed with a Dacron tube or bifurcation graft; in the case of aortic or iliac aneurysm the sac is opened and the graft sutured in. When intra-abdominal surgery is contraindicated, grafts are placed from the ipsilateral axillary or the contralateral common femoral arteries.

Arterial narrowing below the inguinal ligament is bypassed using the long saphenous vein. In its absence a PTFA graft is used and to prolong its patency a collar of vein is interposed between the distal end of the graft and the recipient artery. Aneurysms in the limb are similarly bypassed and are excluded from the circulation to prevent emboli from the clot present within them. Skin perfusion may be improved by lumbar sympathectomy when revascularisation is not feasible.

Clinical and sonographic surveillance is important in monitoring graft patency and impending graft occlusion. With progressive deterioration in symptoms, amputation of the limb should be considered with a planned rehabilitation programme aimed at restoring mobility. This includes physiotherapy and involvement of occupational therapists to ensure that home conditions are appropriate for discharge from hospital.

Examiner's Comments on Answer 1
- *The essay is eminently readable, knowledgeable and concise, with appropriate subdivisions*
- *The introduction defines the problem, gives emphasis to atherosclerosis with its risk factors*
- *Diagnosis is based on the history, examination and investigations, and the candidate has commented on the relevant points in each group*
- *The question is very broad and, therefore, treatment can only be covered in outline. Clear guidelines on each treatment modality are stated*
- *Emphasis is given to the conservative management of most patients, and medical management available is outlined*
- *The importance of angioplasty is given as the first line of management, and the main forms of surgical intervention are summarised*
- *The importance of follow-up is stated*
- *The possible need for amputation is noted, together with the necessary team work for subsequent rehabilitation*

ANSWER 2 – AN ANSWER SHOWING INADEQUATE KNOWLEDGE

The aetiology of chronic arterial disease of the lower limbs is poor general health due to various organic disease states and poor lifestyle. Presentation may be divided into symptoms and signs. The classic symptom of chronic arterial disease of the lower limb is pain. This may be constant or intermittent, and described as affecting mainly the feet or the entire limb, but the most usual presentation is intermittent claudication, this being a sharp pain affecting one or both calves that is induced by exercise and relieved by rest. It is often more troublesome in cold weather. The amount of exercise necessary to bring on the pain is extremely variable but the most troublesome confounding factor in eliciting a history of claudication is the co-existence of osteoarthritis which may make exercise painful and may even mask the presence of arterial disease by precluding walking on its own account. Pain may also arise as a result of ulceration and the patient may complain of cold legs. In late-stage disease a blackened toe may be the presentation. Whilst pain is a feature of ischaemia, tissue which has died is anaesthetic, manipulation of areas of gangrene may cause severe pain at the granulating demarcation between living and dead tissue. Patients with chronic disease may occasionally present acutely, either with a complete cessation of blood flow secondary to thrombus formation, leading to paralysis of the limb which becomes pale, paraesthetic and cold with undetectable pulses or with life-threatening gas gangrene where the patient is systemically ill and the offending limb is pale or green, malodorous and may exhibit the characteristic 'crackling' sensation of gas in the tissues on examination.

Signs of chronic arterial disease of the lower limb include loss of hair, cool skin, ulcers that are characteristically small and well-demarcated, pulses which are difficult or impossible to palpate, blackened extremities and stumps which are sites of previous amputations. The femoral pulses ought always to be auscultated as bruits will often be heard. The management of chronic arterial disease may be divided into investigations, medical and surgical treatment, nursing and physiotherapy. Various radiological investigations may be performed. Such investigations may include angiography, whereas MRI (magnetic resonance imaging) may make a big impact on angiography in the future by allowing digital subtraction images to be constructed non-invasively. Medical treatment will almost always include an anti-clotting agent, such as aspirin, typically 75 mg once daily. Treatment of co-existing medical illness, particularly coronary artery disease should not be overlooked. A number of drugs are available to promote arterial dilation in the peripheries.

Surgical intervention may include endarterectomy if the lesion is relatively localized and in an accessible position. Bypass grafts using PTFE tubing are most useful for restoring blood supply. They may be done at various levels and the femoral–popliteal graft is the classic operation. Surgical treatment often involves amputation if conservative treatment of areas of gangrenous tissue fails. Amputation requires a balance between leaving as much viable tissue as possible and ensuring that the tissue left remains viable; patients are often medically so ill that re-operation is even more undesirable than usual. Nursing care includes care of the whole patient, dressing of ulcers and scrupulous attention to hygiene on areas of tissue which may have died or are of dubious viability. Physiotherapy may improve the function of existing limbs and aid familiarization with artificial limbs, crutches, etc.

Examiner's Comments on Answer 2
Reads well, with many common sense statements, but:
- *Introduction limited to a vague statement, with no mention of risk factors*
- *No sub-headings*
- *Inadquate paragraphs*
- *Too much emphasis given to osteoarthritis and gas gangrene, which have little relevance to the question set*
- *Pain affects the 'entire limb'*
- *Nutrition and postural changes in the foot are missing*
- *No mention of non-invasive tests, viz pressure measurements, imaging or wave-form analysis*
- *No mention of indications for angiography*
- *No mention of drugs, such as anti-platelet agents and their limitations, and PTA – the current first choice of therapeutic measure*
- *No mention of aorto-iliac disease*
- *No mention of extra-anatomic bypass or the limitations of synthetic grafts across the knee*
- *The importance of amputations was mentioned, but no occupational therapy or rehabilitation of the amputee*

SECTION IV:
ESSAY QUESTIONS

ESSAY QUESTIONS

SURGICAL PHYSIOLOGY

1. Discuss the principles of postoperative fluid and electrolyte balance.

2. Describe the preparation of a patient for an abdominal operation and the immediate postoperative management.

3. What is meant by circulatory collapse and shock? List the causes and describe how you would treat one of them.

4. Discuss the investigation and management of a patient who is alleged to have a 'bleeding tendency' before and after major surgery.

TRAUMA AND BURNS

1. A 14-year-old boy is admitted to the Accident and Emergency department with a right-sided abdominal pain after falling 15 feet from a tree. Discuss your assessment and treatment.

2. Describe the priorities of diagnosis and management in a severely injured person.

3. A 10-year-old girl lacerated her wrist on a plate glass window. Describe the structures that may be damaged, indicating how such damage may be diagnosed and treated.

4. Write an essay on the management of skin burns.

5. Discuss the management of a 23-year-old man who was crushed when the seating terrace collapsed at a football stadium.

ORTHOPAEDICS

1. Discuss the management of a 67-year-old woman with osteoarthritis of the hip.

2. A young man was seen in the Orthopaedic clinic with a painful swollen knee following a rotational football injury three days before. Discuss the diagnosis and outline your management.

241

3. Describe the management and potential complications in a 65-year-old woman with a compound fracture of the tibia and fibula.

4. Write an essay on the diagnosis and treatment of fractures of the femur in an adult.

5. An 80-year-old woman complains of pain in her thoracic spine. Discuss the differential diagnoses and the management of the commonest cause of such a symptom.

NEUROSURGERY

1. Write an essay on the assessment and treatment of an adult patient admitted unconscious following a road traffic accident.

2. Describe the various types of peripheral nerve injuries and how you would evaluate and treat them.

3. Describe the common forms of spina bifida and discuss its complications and treatment.

    or

    Write an essay of hydrocephalus and its management.

EYES, ENT AND SKIN

1. Discuss the diagnosis and management of a 36-year-old woman with a malignant melanoma of the skin over her calf.

2. A young man presents to the Accident and Emergency department with discomfort and hazy vision in one eye a few hours after working with a hammer and chisel. What are the possible findings? Discuss the investigations and treatment that may be indicated.

3. Discuss the clinical presentation, the complications and treatment of chronic suppurative otitis media.

4. Describe the causes of a painful red eye and the management of this condition.

5. Describe the causes and discuss the management of a patient with severe nose bleed.

ENDOCRINOLOGY, BREAST AND CHEST

1. Write an essay on the disorders that may arise from abnormalities of the adrenal glands and their surgical treatment.

2. Describe the diagnosis and management of a 40-year-old woman who presents with a solitary nodule in the left lobe of the thyroid.

3. Discuss the diagnosis and management of a 35-year-old woman presenting with a painless lump in the breast.

4. List the causes and discuss the diagnosis and management of a patient with a pneumothorax.

5. Write an essay on the presentation, aetiology, investigation and treatment of a carcinoma of the bronchus.

6. Write an essay on the investigation and interventional and surgical measures used in treating ischaemic heart disease.

UPPER ALIMENTARY TRACT

1. A 64-year-old man presents with a three-month history of increasing difficulty in swallowing solid food. Discuss the diagnosis and management of this patient.

2. Write an essay on the diagnosis and treatment of haematemesis in a 56-year-old woman.

3. Discuss the surgical causes of vomiting in a 14-day-old neonate. Describe how you would diagnose and treat one such condition.

4. Discuss the diagnosis and management of a patient with a perforated peptic ulcer.

5. Write an essay on the indications for splenectomy and the complications of this procedure.

LIVER, GALLBLADDER AND PANCREAS

1. Write an essay on the diagnosis and treatment of a patient suffering from acute cholecystitis.

2. Discuss the presentation, the diagnosis and management of a 68-year-old man with obstructive jaundice.

3. Write an essay on the aetiology, diagnosis and management of acute pancreatitis.

4. Write an essay on portal hypertension and its management.

5. Discuss the causes of liver abscess and its treatment.

SMALL AND LARGE BOWEL

1. Discuss the aetiology and complications of diverticulitis of the colon. Describe the clinical features of the disease and the principles of treatment.

2. Discuss the diagnosis and management of a 32-year-old man who presents with a painful, tender mass in the right iliac fossa.

3. Write an essay on the differential diagnosis and management of a 65-year-old woman complaining of left lower abdominal pain and constipation of 10 weeks' duration.

4. An 18-month-old boy said to be suffering from abdominal colic passed bloodstained mucus per rectum. Discuss the diagnosis and management.

UROLOGY

1. A 35-year-old man presented to the Surgical clinic with a hard, painless swelling of the scrotum. Describe the management of this patient.

2. Describe the management of an adult presenting with haematuria.

3. Describe the types of undescended testis, its treatment and complications.

4. Describe the clinical presentation and management of a patient with a hypernephroma (Grawitz tumour).

5. Write an essay on urethral stricture in an adult male.

VASCULAR SURGERY

1. Describe the causes, presentation and management of an embolus of the femoral artery in a 50-year-old woman seen within six hours of the onset of symptoms.

2. A 61-year-old man presents to the Surgical clinic with a nine-month history of pain in his right calf that occurs after walking 100 yards on the flat, and is relieved by rest. Discuss the diagnosis and management of this patient and the factors that would influence the latter.

3. Discuss the causes and describe the management of gangrene of the toes.

4. Discuss the management of a 70-year-old man presenting with an asymptomatic, pulsatile and expansile mass in the abdomen.

5. Discuss the aetiology and management of lower leg ulceration.

APPENDIX A:
THE FINAL EXAMINATION IN SURGERY

Assessment of clinical competence

Medical training encompasses a wide range of complex and varied activities and has evolved to match the diverse abilities required of the practising clinician. Maintaining these skills is essential for the establishment of professional standards of excellence and satisfying public expectation.

Assessment of clinical competence over such a broad field is fraught with difficulty: it has to examine the results of a number of years of study, covering a large syllabus in a uniform, efficient, competent and reliable fashion. It should ensure that candidates who have achieved the required level of proficiency pass, and those who have not should fail. The examination should be seen by students and examiners as being fair.

The perfect examination not only has to accurately assess knowledge and understanding but also has to evaluate the powers of analysis in problem-solving and decision-making. In the clinical field the candidate's attitude to patients and clinical work, as well as their personal and professional development and conduct, must also be evaluated.

Why examine?

Over the last few decades a number of groups have questioned the need for formal assessment and have proposed continued, faculty-based evaluation in medical education. Nevertheless, the vast majority of medical schools and universities rely on staged examinations to ensure the acquisition of a minimal knowledge base. Satisfactory performance may be accompanied by graduation, certification, and the right to practise. The level of achievement may influence progress and promotion.

Examinations are also valuable for students and teachers to establish personal and departmental standards, and one of the problems of statutory examinations is usually their lack of feedback of the details of a candidate's performance. Internal faculty examinations can be an aid to learning and a means of self-evaluation: this will become of increasing importance with the extension of continued medical education, to help students identify a weakness of personal knowledge and of teaching material. Even the most ardent supporters of continuous assessment cannot deny the stimulus and motivation of an examination, and it does separate good from bad candidates.

246

What system?

To justify their existence examinations have to be seen to be fair and linked with both the training and its stated objectives. Traditional medical examinations have been based on the essay, the oral and the clinical. History and examination are central to a doctor-patient relationship, and the clinical has held its ground in undergraduate and postgraduate assessment (although the division between medicine, surgery and other disciplines has often become blurred, the emphasis being on the history and examination rather than the underlying disorder). Short cases in some schools have been replaced or supplemented by Objective Structured Clinical Examinations (OSCEs) to accompany the written part theory), and orals have been restricted to distinction and borderline candidates.

The essay has come under the greatest scrutiny. Students and examiners have questioned the effectiveness of an essay paper, since the limited number of topics and the possible choices have encouraged students to spot questions and concentrate on only part of the syllabus. The marking of essays is time-consuming and unreliable. There may be variation in an individual examiner's reassessment of papers, as well as between examiners. The variation makes comparison at a national level difficult, and this is further accentuated by what has been described as the deep psychological reluctance of examiners to allocate more than 70% of the total marks allowed for any given essay question.

Attempts to modify the essay included modified essay questions (MEQs), introducing a larger number of questions with a patient vignette, and a variety of sub-sections based on various aspects of diagnosis and treatment. Multiple short answers on a range of topics have also gained favour in some schools. Structured answer questions (SAQs) are a further development of the written assessment, testing problem-solving and decision-making in a structured and objective fashion. They are proving a reliable means of assessing knowledge and understanding in clinical practice.

MCQs also have a wide application in medical assessment, having the potential of covering a wide body of knowledge and, in their extended matched pairs format, introducing reasoned responses rather than item recall. A computerised marking system has eased the examiners' burden in this section. A current trend in the written part of the clinical examination is to include both MCQs and SAQs, the former to determine the candidate's knowledge, and the latter to assess the application of this knowledge by reasoning, interpretation, problem-solving and decision-making.

SAQs

SAQs test the candidate's high-level skills rather than factual recall. They consist of a clinical vignette followed by two to four questions, which may have sub-sections, with an indication of the marks allocated for each correct answer. The choice of scenario is based on common clinical problems pertinent and relevant to the field of study, and covering important concepts and principles relating to the course material. There is no room for trivia, irrelevant or esoteric topics, or interesting rarities.

Clinical information is presented in an ordered fashion, usually describing the history and examination, with or without investigations, of a specific condition. Questions should be clear, unambiguous and requiring the examinee to analyse and make decisions based on the given information. This may involve diagnosis or treatment and may also cover aspects of psychological, social and family history, and ethical issues.

Examiners are given a model answer and a marking schedule that has to be closely adhered to. Marking is time-consuming: allotting a single examiner to each question streamlines the process and allows uniformity of marking for a group of candidates. Any allowances made for near-misses will also be generalised. It is common to double mark a number of scripts to check examiners' inter-observer reliability across the whole examination.

Examiners preparing SAQs should form a panel, draw up a list of topics and allocate these topics among the group. The first draft of each question is read out at a group meeting, and comments made on the content, style, the importance, relevance and its educational standard.

The second draft of the questions is tried on a group of students under examination conditions, noting the time taken to complete 4–8 questions. The answers are analysed and questions again modified if there are obvious misunderstandings, or unexpected ease or difficulty.

Misinterpretation of the stem may lead to an erroneous diagnosis. As the rest of the question is usually based on the stem, a candidate may go off at a tangent in all subsequent answers. The examiners must then make an informed decision in allocating marks for such mishaps, provided the conclusions reached are logical and not far removed from the expected answers. However, in inadequately vetted questions more than one diagnosis may be arrived at from the stem. In such circumstances the onus is firmly on the examiner to accommodate such unanticipated correct responses and mark them fairly.

The completed questions are retained in a question bank. They should be added to each year, attention being given to the choice, number and range of topics. These should match the weighting given to each part of the syllabus. It may take three to five years to build up an adequate bank; after this time any break in security is of less importance.

The stem of a question can often be modified by changing the disease and superficial data, such as the sex, age and timing of the symptoms. This process eases the generation of further questions and allows some degree of comparison of standards when they are being analysed. Questions should be under continuous reappraisal after each use, to assess their performance and discriminatory value. Marks can be influenced by poor quality questions, poor knowledge of answers and errors within the marking system.

Each examination requires 10–12 questions to allow a broad assessment and to produce discriminatory differences between good and bad candidates. Each question used should be independent of the others.

Essays

MCQs are used routinely in most medical qualifying examinations. Nevertheless, medicine is not as black and white as MCQs would suggest, and many brighter students are adverse to this form of assessment. Similarly, although SAQs allow much wider coverage of the syllabus and more objectivity in the marking systems they also restrict the examiner to black or white rigid marking schemes. The limitations of these features are well known to every clinician who has gone over recent examinations with groups of students.

The essay does test a candidate's ability to collect and quantify material, and assesses their powers of original thought and creativity. It determines the candidate's ability to write clear and legible English, and some schools have felt that these qualities should be retained in their assessment. In spite of the expensive manpower required in marking essay questions, an essay does assess a candidate's depth of knowledge in a specified area and, in preparing for an essay paper, candidates have to acquire detailed knowledge of much of the syllabus.

Revision for the essay paper is linked with revision of the whole course. If a candidate's knowledge base is poor, he or she will rightly fail; but, even if it is sound, good examination technique is essential for success. The ease of revision is based on previous knowledge and a good filing system. If disease-based, it is essential to have a checklist for each condition so that current knowledge can be written and then checked against books and stored material to identify deficiencies.

The candidate is expected to have read around topics and patient problems encountered during the clinical course, gaining information from lectures, reviews, and current papers, as well as textbooks. This information should be filed in an easily retrievable form, such as notes in the margins of textbooks, a card system, plenty of lists and clearly written pieces of paper. People vary in the amount of information they can remember at any one time. Any deficiency, however, can be easily reversed during revision, provided previous information was well organised and fully understood at the time it was collected.

Examiners at an undergraduate level are keen to pass candidates, to ensure that they can continue with their careers. However, medical examiners have an obligation to ensure that ignorant and potentially dangerous individuals are not let loose on a patient population. At a postgraduate level examiners have to ensure that a candidate has a comprehensive and in-depth knowledge of their subject: gaps are likely to be penalised.

Regardless of the level of the examination, essays on clinical subjects have a similar format. This is based on an disease or a clinical problem and includes questions on the aetiology, pathology, diagnosis, differential diagnoses, complications, assessment, management and treatment. Each question must be read carefully and every word noted, as they will have been constructed very carefully.

Although the words 'discuss' and a few synonyms imply a certain vagueness, the response must be precise and directed. Having read the question, the answer plan is based on the clinical data required. These will usually correspond to the checklist used to revise each disease.

Diagnosis and differential diagnosis are based on only three sources of information: namely, the **history, examination** and **investigation**. If the diagnosis is given, it may require confirmation from the same three sources. Assessment means diagnosis (history, examination, investigation), but adds the dimension of **severity** of the problems encountered. Management is assessment plus treatment. Although the term may be used loosely, implying just treatment in some questions, it is worth writing a few sentences on confirmation of diagnosis and severity of the problem being treated. Treatment should not be restricted to surgery, as many other problems may require to be sorted out first

Other disciplines that may be involved must be considered, such as nursing, physiotherapy, occupational therapy, and drugs, chemotherapeutic agents and radiotherapy. Radiological intervention forms a major part of treatment in many diseases.

The plan outlining the areas to be covered can be in the answer book or on scrap paper. The plan should take three to six minutes for most essays and allows concentrated thought around the topic. On completion, a line is drawn through it to imply to the examiner that there is more to come, and the first few sentences of the introduction are constructed. This should imply an understanding of the topic, giving the examiner confidence that the essay is on the right track and, hopefully, is of good standard.

There is much debate as to whether headings should be underlined and key words highlighted. This debate is more of a problem to the candidate than the examiner, who is more concerned as to whether the script is legible, and demonstrates knowledge and understanding of the question. Illegibility is an inherent problem with some individuals. Examiners go to considerable effort to give candidates the benefit of the doubt but illegibility can never camouflage ignorance, and candidates would be well advised to write at a rate at which the end product is guaranteed readable to the examiner.

Literacy and mastery of prose are more debatable. As much as examiners would wish medical graduates to be able to write skilfully and coherently, marks are predominantly awarded for factual knowledge and understanding of an essay topic. Success is, therefore, based on an appropriate plan and the development of each heading within it.

Medical schools rarely set regular essays during the clinical course, even when they use this means of final assessment. It is, therefore, appropriate for students who know they will be examined in this way to undertake preliminary practice. A series of essay questions has, therefore, been added after the SAQ sections in each chapter. There is a section on planned structural outlines as a preliminary to writing essays and examples of good and poor answers with examiner's comments. These guidelines may be used to plan and write essays. The relevant practical information will usually be found in the sectional answers and teaching aids, and essays may be swapped with a working partner or discussion group and act as examiners. Subsequently, the plan, development, depth of knowledge, literary style and legibility is discussed. As the finals draw near, the graduation standard becomes apparent, and essays can be accurately assessed by peer review.

Whatever examination system is chosen, it must be reliable, valid and discriminatory, and it should not be influenced by the subjective judgement of an examiner. The examination should be about the contents of a paper and not expertise or prior coaching in the chosen system. Nevertheless, it is essential to have prior exposure to the local examination system and be well versed in its technique. This text is intended to provide that exposure and to educate candidates in the techniques of SAQ and essay writing in the hope of easing their passage to qualification.

APPENDIX B:
SELF-ASSESSMENT SAQ PAPERS

Notes for Readers – SAQ Exam Papers
There are 12 questions in each paper, to be answered in two hours.

- You are advised to spend no more than 10 minutes on each question.
- The questions are designed to promote succinct answers.
- The marks awarded for each section are indicated.

Paper 1: 1.1, 2.1, 3.1, 3.10, 4.1, 5.1, 6.1, 7.1, 8.1, 9.1, 10.1, 11.1

Paper 2: 1.2, 2.2, 3.2, 4.2, 5.2, 6.2, 6.7, 7.2, 8.2, 9.2, 10.2, 11.2

Paper 3: 2.3, 2.11, 3.3, 4.3, 5.3, 6.5, 6.14, 7.3, 8.3, 9.7, 10.3,11.3

Paper 4: 1.3, 2.4, 3.4, 4.4, 5.4, 6.8, 7.4, 8.4, 9.4, 10.4, 10.11,11.5

Paper 5: 1.4, 2.5, 3.5, 4.5, 5.5, 6.3, 7.5, 7.10, 8.5, 9.5, 10.6, 11.6

Paper 6: 1.5, 2.6, 3.6, 4.6, 5.6, 6.6, 6.9, 7.7, 8.6, 9.6, 10.7, 11.7

Paper 7: 1.6, 2.7, 2.13, 3.9, 3.11, 5.7, 6.10, 7.6, 7.8, 8.7, 10.8, 11.8

Paper 8: 1.9, 3.5, 4.3, 5.8, 6.2, 6.12, 7.9, 7.11, 8.8, 10.9, 11.9, 11.11

Paper 9: 1.7, 2.8, 2.10, 3.7, 6.4, 6.13, 7.12, 9.3, 9.9, 10.5, 10.10, 11.12

APPENDIX C:
SELF-ASSESSMENT ESSAY QUESTION PAPERS

Notes for Readers – Essay Exam Papers

There are four questions in each paper, to be answered in two hours.

- You are advised to spend no more than 30 minutes on each question and to spend the first five minutes formulating an outline for your answer.

Paper 1: 2.1, 4.1, 6.1, 8.1

Paper 2: 1.2, 2.2, 9.2, 11.2

Paper 3: 1.2, 2.3, 6.3, 10.3

Paper 4: 2.4, 5.4, 9.4,11.4

Paper 5: 2.5, 5.5, 6.2, 8.2

Paper 6: 1.4, 3.1, 7.1, 10.5

Paper 7: 3.2, 5.3, 7.2, 11.1

Paper 8: 3.3, 4.2, 7.3, 8.3

Paper 9: 3.4, 6.4, 7.4, 10.4

Paper 10: 4.3, 9.3, 10.2, 11.3

Paper 11: 3.5, 5.1, 6.5, 7.5

Paper 12: 1.1, 5.2, 9.1, 10.1

PasTest are the specialists in study guides and revision courses for professional medical qualifications. For 25 years we have been helping doctors to achieve their potential. The new PasTest range of books for medical students includes:

Surgical Finals: Passing the Clinical   £12.25
Kuperberg & Lumley
- 90 examples of favourite long and short surgical cases
- Syllabus checklist for structured revision
- 18 detailed examination schemes with action tables
- 36 tables of differential diagnosis
- 134 popular viva questions for self-assessment
- Recommended reading list and revision index

Medical Finals: Passing the Clinical   £12.25
Moore & Richardson
- 101 typical long cases, short cases and spot diagnoses
- Syllabus checklist for systematic revision
- Vital tips on preparation and presentation
- Structured examination plans for all cases
- Concise teaching notes highlight areas most relevant to finals
- Revision index for easy access to specific topics

Medical Finals: Structured Answer and Essay Questions   £12.25
Feather, Visvanathan & Lumley
- Prepare for the written examination with this unique combination of essay questions and the new structured answer questions
- 141 structured answer questions with detailed teaching notes
- 73 typical essay questions with sample essay plans and model essays
- Invaluable revision checklist to help you to track your progress
- Short textbook reviews enable you to select the best textbooks

All PasTest books are available from good bookshops. For priority mail order service, post or fax the order form overleaf.

Credit card hotline: 01565 755226
E-mail: pastest@dial.pipex.com
Web site: http://ds.dial.pipex.com/pastest

ORDER FORM

Please send me:

☐ One copy of **Surgical Finals: Passing the Clinical**   £12.25
☐ One copy of **Medical Finals: Passing the Clinical**   £12.25
☐ One copy of **Medical Finals: SAQs and Essays**   £12.25

Please add cost of postage:

UK: £1.30 for first book plus 80p for each additional book
Europe: £2.00 for first book plus 80p for each additional book
Outside Europe: £3.50 for first book plus £2.30 for each additional book

Name: ....

Address: ....

....

....

Daytime telephone: ....

☐ I enclose a cheque/money order payable in sterling to PasTest
   Please write your cheque guarantee card number and expiry date
   clearly on the back of your cheque
☐ Please debit my Access/Visa/Switch card

   Card number: ....

   Expiry date: .... Switch Issue Number: ....

Signature: ....

Send this form with your payment to:

**PasTest (Dept UB), Egerton Court, Parkgate Estate,
Knutsford, Cheshire WA16 8DX, UK**

Telephone: 01565 755226 Fax: 01565 650264